MAIN LIBRARY

Bus
50

ACPI

S0-BMG-679

DISCARDED

616.12 Z8F
ZUGIBE, FREDERICK T. 7095442
14 DAYS TO A HEALTHY HEART

DO NOT REMOVE
CARDS FROM POCKET

ALLEN COUNTY PUBLIC LIBRARY

FORT WAYNE, INDIANA 46802

You may return this book to any agency, branch,
or bookmobile of the Allen County Public Library.

DEMCO

14 Days to a Healthy Heart

Other books by Frederick T. Zugibe

Eat, Drink and Lower Your Cholesterol
The Cross and the Shroud:
    A Medical Examiner Investigates the Crucifixion
Diagnostic Histochemistry

14 Days to A

Healthy Heart

FREDERICK T. ZUGIBE, M.D., Ph.D.

7095442

MACMILLAN PUBLISHING COMPANY
NEW YORK
COLLIER MACMILLAN PUBLISHERS
LONDON

Chapter 2

The material in chapter 2 is partially derived from *Exercise And Your Heart,* U.S. Department of Health and Human Services (NIH Publication 81-1677 May 1981, *One Step at a Time, Walking for Exercise and Pleasure* and *Aqua Dynamics,* developed by the President's Council on Fitness and Sports. *Aqua Dynamics* was done in cooperation with the National Spa and Pool Institute. Figures 10, 11, 12 and 13 from L. Zohman, M.D. *Beyond Diets: Exercise Your Way to Fitness and Heart Health,* CPC International, Englewood Cliffs, N.J. Plates 17 and 20, © 1980, Ciba Pharmaceutical Co., Division of Ciba-Geigy Corp. Reprinted with permission from Clinical Symposia, illustrated by Frank Netter, M.D. All rights reserved.

Chapter 4

The material in chapter 4 is largely derived (with permission) from the I Quit program of the American Cancer Society with additional material taken from their Fresh Start program. The Smoker's Self-Awareness Profile as used in the I Quit program was adapted from material provided by the National Clearinghouse for Smoking and Health, Bureau of Health Education, Center for Disease Control, U.S. Dept. of Health, Education and Welfare, Atlanta, Ga. Information was also used from Clearing the Air, developed by the U.S. Dept. of Health and Human Services, Public Health Service, National Institute of Health.

Chapter 5

Part of the sodium information in this chapter is derived from *The Sodium Content of Your Food,* U.S. Dept. of Agriculture, Home and Garden Bulletin #233.

Chapter 6

The Rapid Muscle Relaxation Procedure and diagram are from G. G. Luce and E. Perper "Learning How to Relax" in *Stress* 35: 84–94, 1974, with permission. The Social Readjustment Rating Scale is reprinted from *Journal of Psychosomatic Research* 11: 213–218, 1967, with permission of Dr. T. J. Holmes and Pergamon Press, Ltd.

Appendix

The Metropolitan Height and Weight Tables for Men and Women and How to Determine Your Body Frame by Elbow Breadth were reprinted from *Statistical Bulletin,* January–June 1983, with permission of the Metropolitan Life Insurance Company. The Food Exchange Lists in the Appendix are reprinted from "A Maximal Approach to the Dietary Treatment of the Hyperlipidemias" (from *A Low Cholesterol Diet Manual*) with permission from W. E. Connor, M.D.

Copyright © 1986 by New England Publishing Associates, Inc. and Frederick T. Zugibe

All rights reserved. No part of this book may be reproduced or transmitted in any form or by any means, electronic or mechanical, including photocopying, recording or by any information storage and retrieval system, without permission in writing from the Publisher.

Macmillan Publishing Company
866 Third Avenue, New York, N.Y. 10022
Collier Macmillan Canada, Inc.

Library of Congress Cataloging-in-Publication Data

Zugibe, Frederick T.
  14 days to a healthy heart.

  Bibliography: p. 257.
  Includes index.
  1. Coronary heart disease—Prevention. 2. Coronary heart disease—Diet therapy—Recipes. 3. Heart—Infarction—Prevention. 4. Exercise therapy.
  5. Relaxation. I. Title. II. Title: Fourteen days to a healthy heart.
  RC685.C6Z84 1986   616.1'205   85-8960
  ISBN 0-02-633610-3

Allen County Public Library
Ft. Wayne, Indiana

Macmillan books are available at special discounts for bulk purchases for sales promotions, premiums, fund-raising, or educational use. For details, contact:
  Special Sales Director
  Macmillan Publishing Company
  866 Third Avenue
  New York, N.Y. 10022

10 9 8 7 6 5 4 3 2 1

Printed in the United States of America

Lovingly dedicated to Kitty
for her love, deep faith and inspiration.

This book is not intended as a substitute for the medical advice of physicians. The reader should regularly consult a physician in matters relating to his or her health and particularly in respect to any symptoms that may require diagnosis or medical attention. It is advisable to consult your physician and obtain approval before going on this or any health program.

ACKNOWLEDGMENTS

I am grateful to Elizabeth Frost Knappman for her meticulous editing, keen perception and active participation in this venture; to my editor, Barry Lippman, for his critical evaluation and many important suggestions; to my wife Kitty, for developing most of the recipes and for her moral support; to my daughter Theresa, for calculating the weight reduction diets and caloric values; to my daughter Cathy, for preparing the drawing of the blood pressure apparatus; to Bernadette Abbatecola, for her clerical assistance; to James Costello, for his photographic assistance and ancillary help; and to the many scientists whose contributions have made this book possible.

Contents

Introduction

Every minute of every day 3 Americans will have a heart attack; an alarming 1.5 million people a year. Of these, 555,000 will die.

It was not always like this. At the beginning of this century, heart disease accounted for only 10 percent of all deaths. This rate gradually increased over the years until in the 1960s it reached a startling 39 percent. But between 1968 and 1977, as a result of changes in our life-style, there was an unexpected decline in the number of deaths from heart attacks and strokes. Millions of Americans stopped smoking, started jogging and reduced the amount of cholesterol-rich foods in their diets. In addition, doctors began using new methods in blood pressure control to treat their patients. But despite these improvements, heart attack is still our number-one killer. And it is discouraging to me both as a cardiologist and as a medical examiner to see so many men and women in their prime dying of this disease. Since an important role of the medical examiner—one that is not usually appreciated—is to identify factors in order to prevent needless deaths, I felt a compelling need to write this book.

14 Days to a Healthy Heart is for people like you who want to prevent a heart attack. It contains a practical drug-free program that will let anyone—in just fourteen days—learn a lifetime pattern that can eliminate or modify the risks of heart attack and related diseases.

14 Days to a Healthy Heart is an integrated plan of sound nutrition, stress management, nonsmoking conditioning and aerobic exercise, all designed to fit easily and pleasantly into your most crowded days.

Now, in just fourteen days, you can lower your blood cholesterol level, LDL-cholesterol (bad cholesterol) and triglyceride levels and raise your HDL (good cholesterol), all without using drugs.

In just fourteen days most people with high blood pressure can lower their pressure to normal or to a lower level without drugs. High blood pressure is a major risk factor that has been dubbed "the silent killer."

In just fourteen days you can learn to manage your stress more successfully. Unmanageable stress can lead to clogged arteries, excess weight, heavy smoking and elevated blood pressure, greatly increasing your chances of suffering a heart attack.

In just fourteen days you who are habitual smokers can kick the smoking habit. Smoking lowers HDL-cholesterol (good cholesterol), elevates blood pressure and increases the risk of heart attack.

In just fourteen days you can lose an average of four to eight pounds healthfully. Obesity is an important risk factor greatly influencing other risk factors.

In just fourteen days you can learn a lifetime pattern for eliminating the risks of heart attack and related diseases that strike so many people, including young adults and children.

My fourteen-day plan could save your heart, starting today, and add healthful and vigorous years to your life.

> *The health of the people is really the foundation upon which all their happiness and all their powers as a state depend.*
>
> *—Benjamin Disraeli*

14 Days to a Healthy Heart

Chapter One

How a Heart Attack

Occurs: The New

Medical Scenario

The heart is an amazing pump built to last a life-time—just exactly.

—Anonymous

Before introducing the fourteen-day plan for a healthier heart, let me briefly explain how the heart works and how and why a heart attack occurs.

THE HEART

The heart is a pump that forces blood through a vast network of arteries to all parts of the body. Operating with greater efficiency than any machine, the heart beats over 100,000 times each day without stopping and pumps about 4,500 gallons of blood through more than 60,000 miles of vessels to deliver oxygen and nutrients to the cells of the body.

The bulk of the heart is made up of a muscle called the *myocardium*, lined on the inside and outside with elongated cells and support tissue.

Heart Attack

The heart receives its oxygen and nutrients through two main blood vessels, the *left* and *right coronary arteries*. If any of these arteries or its branches becomes blocked or narrowed so that the blood cannot get

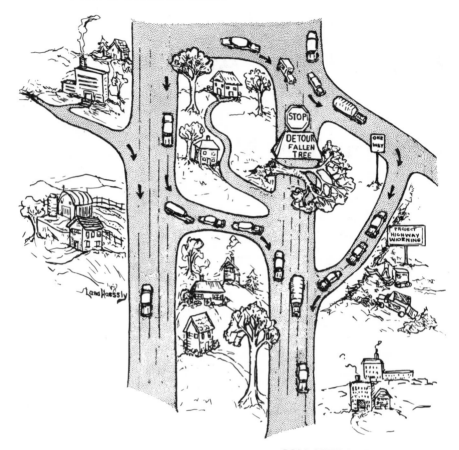

COLLATERAL CIRCULATION

through, areas of the heart muscle beyond the blockage will die. This is called a *heart attack*. The heart muscle that dies is called an *infarct*. Thus the term *myocardial infarction* is a synonym for a heart attack (a stroke is caused by a similar blockage in the arteries of the brain).

The blockage in a heart attack is almost always caused by a complex disease process in which fatty substances are deposited within the artery wall, progressively narrowing the passage. The deposit, referred to as a *plaque* or *atheroma* (from the Greek word *atheros*, meaning "porridge"), contains cholesterol, fats, calcium and other substances. This condition is called *atherosclerosis*. Further, a blood clot sometimes forms in an area partly blocked by a plaque; this is known as a *coronary thrombosis*—an often fatal complication of atherosclerosis.

WHO SURVIVES?

About 20 percent of heart attacks are fatal—but why do some people die and others live? The ability to survive depends on several factors. First and foremost is the extent of a person's *collaterals*—extra blood vessels that go around the areas of blockage in a manner similar to the way side streets bypass main thoroughfares (illus. 1). For example, if a major highway that services a city is blocked by a large tree across the road, it would be difficult to bring food products and other necessities into the city. If, however, there are side roads, the traffic can easily be detoured by way of these side roads to bring in the necessary items. If extra vessels are lacking in the person who suffers a coronary blockage, then not enough oxygen can reach the heart tissues. This can promote a serious rhythm disturbance (ventricular fibrillation) that can cause the heart to stop. This is known as a *cardiac arrest*.

CAUSES OF HEART ATTACK

The answer to the question of what causes heart attacks is very simple— no one really knows. In spite of recent discoveries in the field of heart research, the specific cause of the disease process causing a heart attack is not fully understood. However, heart scientists have identified the following risk factors, which have been implicated in causing heart attacks:

1. high blood cholesterol
2. low levels of good cholesterol (HDL-cholesterol) and high levels of bad cholesterol (LDL-cholesterol)
3. cigarette smoking
4. high blood pressure
5. lack of physical activity
6. heredity
7. obesity
8. stress
9. diabetes
10. oral contraceptives

High Blood Cholesterol

Cholesterol is a fatty substance found only in animal tissue, never in plants. Cholesterol serves a useful function in transporting fats, in producing hormones and in making nerve cells. Yet the general public knows cholesterol only as a harbinger of heart attacks. This is because in the late 1950s scientists participating in the world-famous Massachusetts-based Framingham study reported that individuals with high blood cholesterol levels suffered three times as many heart attacks as those with low cholesterol levels. This established a connection between high cholesterol levels in the blood and the development of heart attacks. Further, in those nations where heart attack is the number-one killer, the cholesterol levels are very high, and in those nations where heart attacks are rare, the cholesterol levels are low. Today more than forty million Americans have moderate to high blood cholesterol levels.

WHAT CONSTITUTES HIGH BLOOD CHOLESTEROL LEVEL?

Reports from Framingham in 1977 and the Pooling Project Research Group in 1978 showed that the majority of heart attacks occurred among people who had in the range of 220 to 260 milligrams of cholesterol in about every 3⅓ ounces of blood. Top experts in the field consider levels between 200 to 220 to be normal; an increased risk is associated with rising levels above this range.

Although most scientists accept the association of elevated cholesterol levels with an increased risk of heart attacks, there has been considerable controversy as to whether lowering the blood cholesterol will reduce the risk. It will, according to a ten-year study sponsored by the National Heart, Lung and Blood Institute, which announced its findings in 1984. This study involved 3,806 men between the ages of thirty-five and fifty-nine with blood cholesterol levels of 265 or higher. The results clearly demonstrated that the risk of coronary disease can be reduced by lowering blood cholesterol and that the bigger the drop in cholesterol, the lower the incidence of heart attacks. The recommendation of this study: try a dietary approach first, but if it is unsuccessful; then have your physician try drugs.

GOOD AND BAD CHOLESTEROL

Until recently scientists considered all cholesterol undesirable. Then they began to look at substances called *lipoproteins*. These are proteins that combine with cholesterol so that the latter can be transported in the blood. Here the researchers discovered gold; they found that there were two types of lipoprotein that, when attached to cholesterol, were more important in predicting heart attacks than the blood cholesterol level: the *low-*

density lipoprotein cholesterol (LDL, or bad cholesterol) and the *high-density lipoprotein* cholesterol (HDL, or good cholesterol). Bad cholesterol transports and deposits the cholesterol in the artery walls. Good cholesterol acts like a scavenger, removing cholesterol from the walls of arteries and depositing it in safe areas. From 1968 to 1972 the Framingham Study followed 2,815 men and women forty-nine to eighty-two years of age. They found that the lower the good cholesterol in the blood, the greater the risk of a heart attack, angina and sudden death. The higher the good cholesterol, the less the risk. Conversely, the more bad cholesterol in the blood, the greater the risk of a heart attack, angina and sudden death, the lower the bad cholesterol, the lower the risk.

After this discovery a flurry of studies revealed impressive results. All the following risk factors were shown to reduce significantly the levels of good cholesterol in the blood: smoking, obesity, oral contraceptives, diabetes and high-saturated-fat diets. Interestingly, aerobic exercise, weight reduction and the estrogens raised the levels of good cholesterol. One to two drinks of alcoholic beverages may also raise the good cholesterol.

This major breakthrough is also important because it enables us to screen high-risk people by means of a simple blood test. A good cholesterol level below 35 milligrams per 3⅓ ounces of blood means a high risk for heart disease. A value above 55 means a low risk. There is a minor variation in the values for women, which are slightly higher.

TRIGLYCERIDES

The triglycerides are the visible fats in various foods. They are also present in the blood and in the fat storage areas of the body. The blood triglycerides are derived from the fatty foods in our meals but are also produced from various carbohydrates in the diet and from alcoholic beverages. While elevated blood triglycerides are not considered to be an independent risk factor, they are related to the occurrence of heart disease in some persons and therefore should be reduced. These substances are frequently elevated in untreated diabetics and in obese individuals and can be measured by a simple laboratory test.

Cigarette Smoking

Cigarette smoking is like a tornado that leaves nothing but devastation in its wake. It causes a great number of diseases, from emphysema to cancer. But the link with heart disease has been the most dramatic. In fact, many consider cigarette smoking as one of the key risk factors in heart attacks. In a long-term study of thirty-nine- to fifty-nine-year-old male cigarette smokers and nonsmokers, the risk of heart disease was twice as great for the smokers as for the nonsmokers, and the risk was more than three times as great for heavy smokers. However, cigar and pipe smokers faced a risk no different from that of nonsmokers.

The manner in which cigarette smoking causes heart attacks is not fully known. Yet it seems partly due to an ability to lower the good cholesterol. When the good cholesterol is lowered by smoking, neither exercise, diet nor other factors usually known to raise it can do so any longer. Further, blood clots faster and makes a tougher clot after only one cigarette. This fact is especially important in light of two recent independent large-scale studies that reported higher death rates from coronary thrombosis in heavy smokers. Finally, carbon monoxide, which deprives red blood corpuscles of oxygen, can be 15 percent higher in the blood of smokers. This is of particular significance in individuals with narrowed coronary arteries. In addition to the role of cigarettes as a risk factor in coronary artery disease and heart attacks, a recent study reported in 1984 showed an association of smoking with heart muscle disease (cardiomyopathy). A word of caution: "safe" cigarettes do not lower the incidence of heart attacks; neither do they reduce carbon monoxide levels in the blood.* Moreover smoking appears to alter the absorption of ascorbic acid (vitamin C), which has been reported to raise the good cholesterol and lower the bad cholesterol and triglycerides.

High Blood Pressure

High blood pressure, or hypertension, afflicts 1 out of every 4 Americans. A staggering 37,330,000 adults have the disease, and every year about 31,800 of them die. Most people are totally unaware that they have high blood pressure and usually discover it during a routine physical examination at work or at a blood pressure screening program.

The risk of coronary disease for people with high blood pressure is three to four times that of their contemporaries. Moreover, actuarial studies of approximately five million people made by twenty-five large insurance

---

*The term "safe" cigarettes refers to the use of filters that allegedly remove more of the tars and nicotine, resulting in a low-nicotine cigarette. A ten-year study at the Framingham Project of individuals using filter cigarettes failed to reveal a decrease in coronary heart disease, and the use of these low-tar filters had no effect on reducing the carbon monoxide levels.

companies confirmed that mortality rises with increasing elevation of blood pressure. And the report of the United States Veterans Administration Cooperative Study Group published in the *Journal of the American Medical Association* in 1970 showed a definite reduction in mortality in treated versus untreated individuals with high blood pressure.

When high blood pressure is present along with diabetes, obesity, cigarette smoking, elevated serum cholesterol or birth control pills, the total cardiac risk multiplies precipitously. Oral contraceptives have also been shown to cause high blood pressure. Finally, blacks have a higher incidence of high blood pressure, with about one out of every four people affected. (They may have a genetic inability to handle salt.)

There is a definite link between the use of salt and high blood pressure in some men and women. The Japanese, who consume large amounts of salted fish and soy sauce, both of which are very high in sodium chloride, have the highest incidence of high blood pressure in the world. And Eskimos, who eat a low level of salt, are practically free of high blood pressure. The moral of this story is that if you are an inveterate salt user, it is important that you shake the habit.

Lack of Physical Activity

Physically inactive people have about two times the risk of having a heart attack as do active men and women. This was first shown in a landmark study of conductors and drivers of London double-decker buses in 1953. The drivers, who sat down all day, had twice as many heart attacks as the conductors, who had to climb up and down the stairs between the decks. Moreover, a famous twenty-two-year study of 6,351 San Francisco Bay area longshoremen in 1975 showed a marked decrease in the coronary death rate in people with high levels of vigorous physical activity. A long-term study published in 1984 involving 16,936 male Harvard alumni ages thirty-five through eighty-four showed almost twice as many deaths from cardiovascular disease in the sedentary groups as there were in the most active groups using 2,000 or more calories each week in walking, jogging, sports play and the like.

The ability to survive a heart attack is also greater for active than sedentary people. This was strikingly demonstrated in a classic 1966 study of 55,000 Greater New York men between the ages of twenty-five and sixty-four. Of 301 first heart attacks recorded, only 17 percent of the most active died, as compared to 49 percent of the least active. There are several reasons for this: increased physical activity raises the good cholesterol and lowers the bad cholesterol and triglycerides; it also lowers blood pressure, aids in weight loss and causes a rise in certain chemicals in the body called *fibrinolysins*, which dissolve blood clots. Exercise also promotes the development of collateral blood vessels.

Heredity

Heart disease occurs more frequently in some families than in others. It is also four times more prevalent in brothers or sisters of victims of coronary atherosclerosis than in siblings of people without the disease.

Does this mean we inherit heart disease—that our genes "say" heart attack? Not at all. The close association observed could just as well be due to the fact that families usually have the same type of diet and develop similar life patterns that cause them to avoid physical activity, to smoke cigarettes or to react to stress in the same way. Yes, heredity is an independent risk factor, but we don't "inherit" a heart attack. What we may inherit are certain defects that lead to heart attack, such as an abnormality in cholesterol metabolism or a type of coronary artery that has a tendency to develop atherosclerosis under various environmental conditions. Therefore, if Pat Brown is born with a coronary artery similar to that of his father who died of a heart attack, he may develop the disease if he is exposed to the various risk factors.

The oft-repeated statement that nothing can be done about heredity is basically true; however, something can be done to modify its effects. For example, if a woman has inherited skin that is extremely sensitive to an ingredient contained in a certain brand of soap, she cannot change her skin but she can change soaps. The more risk factors we can eliminate, the less important heredity becomes.

Obesity

Scientists have long debated whether obesity causes heart disease or whether the increased risk is instead related to the higher incidence of high blood pressure, diabetes and elevated blood fats and cholesterol in overweight people. Life insurance studies have shown a higher incidence of cardiovascular disease in overweight individuals as compared to the rest of the population, resulting in overweight policyholders paying higher premiums. But recently these studies have been questioned, because it was discovered that the small percentage of overweight individuals who opted to pay higher premiums did not represent the percentage of similarly overweight people in the general population. Nonetheless, a definite association exists between coronary artery disease and excessive degrees of obesity or any degree of obesity in people with high blood pressure, diabetes or high blood cholesterol and triglycerides. In February of 1985 a panel of experts convened by the National Institute of Health released a statement strongly advising anyone 20 percent or more overweight to lose weight. They further emphasized that the location of the fat deposits must also be considered since new research shows that abdominal fat is dangerous and closely linked to heart disease and diabetes while other locations such as fat on the hips may be innocuous. Some authorities now only consider weight 10 percent above a person's average as a risk. But anyone with high blood pressure, a high triglyceride level or diabetes, even if only a few pounds overweight, should start a reducing program.

Stress

Stress is the way the body responds physically and mentally to the demands of everyday living. It may be lifesaving or death-producing, depending on the circumstances.

During an emergency situation, in which there is a threat of danger or harm, such as running for your life from an assailant, a primitive alarm system is alerted in the body that triggers a "fight or flight" reaction: heart rate increases, blood pressure rises, respiratory rate increases, sugar is poured into the circulation, pupils enlarge, senses become sharper and the blood flow to muscles increases. After the danger is overcome, by fighting or fleeing, the alarm is turned off and things begin to return to normal.

Now how does this apply to heart attacks? In primitive times, when a fight-or-flight reaction was evoked by danger, the cave dweller would either fight or flee, thereby dissipating the effects of stress. In modern times, instead of danger, this reaction is precipitated by job tensions, awesome responsibilities, corporate pressures, economic pressures, inflation, anxiety, job insecurity, divorce suits, child custody battles, ego threats and the like. But, unlike what happened to our ancestors, the alarm system becomes jammed. It is not turned off by fighting or fleeing, because the person can't fight back (by punching the boss, quitting her job, etc.). Therefore, the fight-or-flight reaction continues in an unrelenting manner for anywhere from days to years, taking its toll on the cardiovascular system.

One specific behavior pattern dubbed the *type A personality* may be related to an increased incidence of heart attack. This pattern is characterized by aggressiveness, competitiveness, a need to excel, hostility, a driving personality and speech explosiveness. People with these characteristics have trouble relaxing when they are away from their jobs, appear very tense, and eat, speak, drive and work in a fast manner. They are also impatient in traffic, pound tables and are irritable when waiting on line. Type A workers have two times the chance of developing a heart attack than do type Bs (people who do not share these characteristics).

Stress is not dangerous and may even have a good effect if a person is in complete control of the situation. Top executives who make important decisions have the least risk of a heart attack. Their underlings suffer more because they are not in control of their work. In 1974 the Metropolitan Life Insurance Company studied more than a thousand executive men taken from the Fortune 500 companies and found that these top-echelon males had a 37-percent lower mortality rate than a comparable group of males in other positions. The ability to control one's own life has beneficial effects. But a life that is controlled by others results in untold stress on the cardiovascular system.

Diabetes

Diabetes mellitus is a disease that prevents our bodies from properly using the sugars and starches we eat. People with diabetes suffer from more heart attacks and at an earlier age and have more coronary artery disease than people who do not have this condition. Five to six times as many heart attacks occur in men and women under forty-five with diabetes as in those who do not have the disease. About 75 percent of diabetics with overt disease die of the complications of atherosclerosis.

A diabetic cannot use blood sugar for energy, either because he does not produce enough of the right kind of insulin or because his body cannot use its insulin properly. The association of diabetes with heart attacks is not fully understood. But it may be related to elevations in cholesterol and blood fats (triglycerides and bad cholesterol) and to the stimulation by insulin of certain cells in the artery wall to start the atherosclerosis process. Diabetics in other areas of the world, such as Japan, the Middle East, and North Africa, have no increased risk of heart attack, indicating that diabetes is not a primary factor in causing heart attacks but must augment other risk factors. Risk factors such as obesity multiply the effects of diabetes, while increased physical activity decreases it.

Birth Control Pills

A woman has a four-times-greater risk of having a heart attack if she uses birth control pills than if she doesn't, according to a 1976 Boston University study. This risk rises astronomically if she is a heavy cigarette smoker or has any other risk factors, such as high blood pressure, obesity, diabetes or elevated blood cholesterol. In women on birth control pills who are also heavy smokers, the risk of a heart attack jumps to twenty times that of a nonsmoker who is not on the pill.

We don't know how birth control pills cause heart attacks. But it may be because they elevate the bad cholesterol in the blood and reduce the good cholesterol, thereby promoting atherosclerosis in the arteries. Since birth control pills interfere with the clotting process, they may cause a heart attack by forming a blood clot in a coronary artery. These pills are also known to cause high blood pressure in some women.

YOUR HEART ATTACK RISK PROFILE

The following test, called Risko, was developed by the Michigan and the American Heart Associations as a heart hazard appraisal. Based on the Framingham, Stanford and Chicago heart disease studies, it concentrates on five of the major heart-attack-risk factors: obesity, high blood pressure, elevated blood cholesterol, cigarette smoking and birth control pill use. Your score will be even higher if you have any of the other risk factors that were previously discussed.

Your Risko score becomes less accurate when using the weight category to estimate your blood pressure or blood cholesterol. This can be corrected and made more accurate by having your physician determine these two values for you.

The score is an indicator of real risk for men over thirty-five and women over forty-five but reflects an upper limit on the true risk for men under thirty-five and women under forty-five. The real risk is probably lower than that indicated by the score in the latter age group.

Risko:

MEN

Find the column for your age group. Everyone
starts with a score of 10 points. Work down the
page *adding* points to your score or *subtracting*
points from your score.

1. Weight
Locate your weight category in the table on the next page.
If you are in . . .

	54 or younger	55 or older
	STARTING SCORE $\boxed{10}$	STARTING SCORE $\boxed{10}$
weight category A	Subtract 2	Subtract 2
weight category B	Subtract 1	Add 0
weight category C	Add 1	Add 1
weight category D	Add 2	Add 3
	Equals ☐	**Equals** ☐

2. Systolic blood pressure
Use the "first" or "higher" number from your most recent blood pressure measurement. If you do not know your blood pressure, estimate it by using the letter for your weight category. If your blood pressure is . . .

A	119 or less	Subtract 1	Subtract 5
B	between 120 and 139	Add 0	Subtract 2
C	between 140 and 159	Add 0	Add 1
D	160 or greater	Add 1	Add 4
		Equals ☐	**Equals** ☐

3. Blood cholesterol level
Use the number from your most recent blood cholesterol test. If you do not know your blood cholesterol, estimate it by using the letter for your weight category. If your blood cholesterol is . . .

A	199 or less	Subtract 2	Subtract 1
B	between 200 and 224	Subtract 1	Subtract 1
C	between 225 and 249	Add 0	Add 0
D	250 or higher	Add 1	Add 0
		Equals ☐	**Equals** ☐

4. Cigarette smoking

If you . . .

(If you smoke a pipe, but not cigarettes, use the same score adjustment as those cigarette smokers who smoke less than a pack a day.)

A	do not smoke	Subtract 1	Subtract 2
B	smoke less than a pack a day	Add 0	Subtract 1
C	smoke a pack a day	Add 1	Add 0
D	smoke more than a pack a day	Add 2	Add 3

Final score equals ☐   **Final score equals** ☐

Weight Table for Men

Look for your height (without shoes) in the far left column and then read across to find the category into which your weight (in indoor clothing) would fall.

YOUR HEIGHT FT	IN	WEIGHT CATEGORY (lbs.) A	B	C	D	
5	1	up to 123	124-148	149-173	174 plus	Because both
5	2	up to 126	127-152	153-178	179 plus	blood pressure
5	3	up to 129	130-156	157-182	183 plus	and blood cho-
5	4	up to 132	133-160	161-186	187 plus	lesterol are re-
5	5	up to 135	136-163	164-190	191 plus	lated to weight,
5	6	up to 139	140-168	169-196	197 plus	an estimate of
5	7	up to 144	145-174	175-203	204 plus	these risk fac-
5	8	up to 148	149-179	180-209	210 plus	tors for each
5	9	up to 152	153-184	185-214	215 plus	weight category
5	10	up to 157	158-190	191-221	222 plus	is printed at the
5	11	up to 161	162-194	195-227	228 plus	bottom of the
6	0	up to 165	166-199	200-232	233 plus	table.
6	1	up to 170	171-205	206-239	240 plus	
6	2	up to 175	176-211	212-246	247 plus	
6	3	up to 180	181-217	218-253	254 plus	
6	4	up to 185	186-223	224-260	261 plus	
6	5	up to 190	191-229	230-267	268 plus	
6	6	up to 195	196-235	236-274	275 plus	
Estimate of systolic blood pressure		**119 or less**	**120 to 139**	**140 to 159**	**160 or more**	
Estimate of blood cholesterol		**199 or less**	**200 to 224**	**225 to 249**	**250 or more**	

NOTE: Reproduced with permission of American Heart Association.

Risko:

WOMEN

Find the column for your age group. Everyone
starts with a score of 10 points. Work down the
page *adding* points to your score or *subtracting*
points from your score.

1. Weight
Locate your weight category in the table on the next page.
If you are in . . .

		54 or younger	55 or older
		STARTING SCORE [10]	STARTING SCORE [10]
☐	weight category A	Subtract 2	Subtract 2
☐	weight category B	Subract 1	Subtract 1
☐	weight category C	Add 1	Add 0
☐	weight category D	Add 2	Add 1
		Equals ☐	**Equals** ☐

2. Systolic blood pressure
Use the "first" or "higher" number from your most recent blood pressure measurement. If you do not know your blood pressure, estimate it by using the letter for your weight category. If your blood pressure is . . .

		54 or younger	55 or older
A	119 or less	Subtract 2	Subtract 3
B	between 120 and 139	Subtract 1	Add 0
C	between 140 and 159	Add 0	Add 3
D	160 or greater	Add 1	Add 6
		Equals ☐	**Equals** ☐

3. Blood cholesterol level
Use the number from your most recent blood cholesterol test. If you do not know your blood cholesterol, estimate it by using the letter for your weight category. If your blood cholesterol is . . .

		54 or younger	55 or older
A	199 or less	Subtract 1	Subtract 3
B	between 200 and 224	Add 0	Subtract 1
C	between 225 and 249	Add 0	Add 1
D	250 or higher	Add 1	Add 3
		Equals ☐	**Equals** ☐

4. Cigarette smoking
If you . . .

	54 or younger	55 or older
☐ do not smoke	Subtract 1	Subtract 2
☐ smoke less than a pack a day	Add 0	Subtract 1
☐ smoke a pack a day	Add 1	Add 1
☐ smoke more than a pack a day	Add 2	Add 4
	Equals ☐	**Equals** ☐

5. Estrogen use (See Author Comment below.)

*Birth control pills and hormone drugs contain estrogen. A few examples are: *Premarin *Ogan *Menstranol *Provera *Evex *Menest *Estinyl *Meurium*

*Have you ever taken estrogen for five or more years in a row?
*Are you age 35 years or older and are now taking estrogen?

No to both questions	Add 0	Add 0
Yes to one or both questions	Add 1	Add 3

Final score equals ☐   Final score equals ☐

Author Comment: Middle age and older post menopausal women should omit Category #5 since recent studies indicate relatively no association between coronary heart disease and estrogen use in this age group.

Weight Table for Women

Look for your height (without shoes) in the far left column and then read across to find the category into which your weight (in indoor clothing) would fall.

YOUR HEIGHT FT IN	WEIGHT CATEGORY (lbs.) A	B	C	D	
4 8	up to 101	102-122	123-143	144 plus	Because both
4 9	up to 103	104-125	126-146	147 plus	blood pressure
4 10	up to 106	107-128	129-150	151 plus	and blood cho-
4 11	up to 109	110-132	133-154	155 plus	lesterol are re-
5 0	up to 112	113-136	137-158	159 plus	lated to weight,
5 1	up to 115	116-139	140-162	163 plus	an estimate of
5 2	up to 119	120-144	145-168	169 plus	these risk fac-
5 3	up to 122	123-148	149-172	173 plus	tors for each
5 4	up to 127	128-154	155-179	180 plus	weight category
5 5	up to 131	132-158	159-185	186 plus	is printed at the
5 6	up to 135	136-163	164-190	191 plus	bottom of the
5 7	up to 139	140-168	169-196	197 plus	table.
5 8	up to 143	144-173	174-202	203 plus	
5 9	up to 147	148-178	179-207	208 plus	
5 10	up to 151	152-182	183-213	214 plus	
5 11	up to 155	156-187	188-218	219 plus	
6 0	up to 159	160-191	192-224	225 plus	
6 1	up to 163	164-196	197-229	230 plus	
Estimate of systolic blood pressure	119 or less	120 to 139	140 to 159	160 or more	
Estimate of blood cholesterol	199 or less	200 to 224	225 to 249	250 or more	

WHAT YOUR SCORE MEANS

0-4 | You have one of the lowest risks of heart disease for your age and sex.

5-9 | You have a low to moderate risk of heart disease for your age and sex but there is some room for improvement.

10-14 | You have a moderate to high risk of heart disease for your age and sex, with considerable room for improvement on some factors.

15-19 | You have a high risk of developing heart disease for your age and sex with a great deal of room for improvement on all factors.

20 & over | You have a very high risk of developing heart disease for your age and sex and should take immediate action on all risk factors.

WARNING

*If you have diabetes, gout or a family history of heart disease, your actual risk will be greater than indicated by this appraisal.

*If you do not know your current blood pressure or blood cholesterol level, you should visit your physician or health center to have them measured. Then figure your score again for a more accurate determination of your risk.

*If you are overweight, have high blood pressure or high blood cholesterol, or smoke cigarettes, your long-term risk of heart disease is increased even if your risk in the next several years is low.

HOW TO REDUCE YOUR RISK

*Try to quit smoking permanently. There are many programs available.

*Have your blood pressure checked regularly, preferably every twelve months after age 40. If your blood pressure is high, see your physician. Remember, blood pressure medicine is only effective if taken regularly.

*Consider your daily exercise (or lack of it). A half hour of brisk walking, swimming or other enjoyable activity should not be difficult to fit into your day.

*Give some serious thought to your diet. If you are overweight, or eat a lot of foods high in saturated fat or cholesterol (whole milk, cheese, eggs, butter, fatty foods, fried foods), then changes should be made in your diet. Look for the *American Heart Association Cookbook* at your local bookstore.

*Visit or write your local Heart Association for further information and copies of free pamphlets on many related subjects including:

• Reducing your risk of heart attack.
• Controlling high blood pressure.
• Eating to keep your heart healthy.
• How to stop smoking.
• Exercising for good health.

SOME WORDS OF CAUTION

*If you have diabetes, gout, or a family history of heart disease, your real risk of developing heart disease will be greater than indicated by your RISKO score. If your score is high and you have one or more of these additional problems, you should give particular attention to reducing your risk.

*If you are a woman under 45 years or a man under 35 years of age, your RISKO score represents an upper limit on your real risk of developing heart disease. In this case your real risk is probably lower than indicated by your score.

*If you are a woman whose use of estrogen has contributed to a high RISKO score, you may want to consult your physician. Do not automatically discontinue your prescription.

*Using your weight category to estimate your systolic blood pressure or your blood cholesterol level makes your RISKO score less accurate.

 • Your score will tend to overestimate your risk if your actual values on these two important factors are average for someone of your height and weight.

 • our score will underestimate your risk if your actual blood pressure or cholesterol level is above average for someone of your height or weight.

Chapter Two

Your 14-Day Heart-Saving

Exercise Plan

The wise, for cure, on exercise depend;
God never made his work for man to mend.
                              —John Dryden

Cardiovascular fitness is a physical state in which a person can exercise at a high level of activity with great efficiency. The means that the cardiovascular system copes with physical and emotional activities at a low heart rate, with low blood pressure and with less fatigue. There is thus less strain on the cardiovascular system.

Cardiac conditioning is dependent on rhythmic acceleration of the heart rate. Therefore, exercises that improve cardiovascular conditioning must be performed in a continuous repetitive motion for sustained periods. These are called *aerobic exercises*, because blood flow is continuously increased througout the circulatory system, providing oxygen to the heart and muscles. The aerobic exercises include walking, jogging, stationary cycling, swimming, jumping rope, trampoline routines and cross-country skiing.

Many exercises are performed daily both at home and in gyms throughout the world that are excellent for increasing muscle strength or skill in performance but have no beneficial effect on cardiovascular fitness. One type, known as *isometric* exercises, has no place in cardiac conditioning programs, since they may increase the blood pressure to dangerous levels or cause an undue strain on the heart. They include weight lifting, dynamic tension, shot putting, chin-ups, sit-ups, arm wrestling, snow shoveling and the like. The second type is exercise that improves coordination, skill and muscle tone after the person has learned and practices certain movement patterns. Although these exercises are enjoyable, they do not condition the heart, because they are not vigorous and sustained. These include baseball, soccer, bowling, golf, football, softball, volleyball, playing musical instruments and so on.

HEALTH CHECK TEST

The following test will determine whether you must see a doctor before exercising. If you answer yes to *any* of the following questions, you must have a complete physical examination, including a cardiac stress test, before starting the exercise program. Many experts, however, recommend that anyone over thirty-five years of age should have a physical examination before beginning an exercise program.

HEALTH CHECK TEST

☐ Have you ever had a heart attack?
☐ Do you have a heart murmur?
☐ Do you have high blood pressure?
☐ Do you have angina pectoris?
☐ Do you have spells of fainting or dizziness?
☐ Do you experience pain or chest pressure or discomfort in the chest, down the left arm, left shoulder, jaw or neck after mild exertion?
☐ Do you experience these symptoms in cold air, after a heavy meal or with anxiety?
☐ Do you experience shortness of breath (breathlessness) after mild exertion, in cold air, after a meal or with anxiety?
☐ Do you take nitroglycerin or any pill under the tongue for chest pain?
☐ Do you take other drugs or wear a chest patch for chest pain or any heart condition?
☐ Do you get cramps in your legs when you walk a short distance (a few blocks)?
☐ Do you have a strong family history of heart disease in individuals under 50–60 years of age?
☐ Do you have diabetes?
☐ Are you overweight at more than 20–25 pounds?
☐ Do you have any pain?
☐ Do you experience any nausea after exertion?
☐ Do you get heart palpitations?
☐ Do you have a rhythm disturbance of your heart including a rapid heart?
☐ Do you smoke heavily (one or more packs/day)?
☐ Did you doctor ever tell you that your heart was enlarged or your electrocardiogram was abnormal?
☐ Did you ever have an abnormal stress test?

☐ Do you have arthritis or other bone or joint problems, such as gout?
☐ Do you have lung disease, such as emphysema, bronchitis or asthma?
☐ Do you have any kidney disease or gout?
☐ Do you have any other significant disease?

BEGINNING THE 14-DAY HEART-SAVING EXERCISE PROGRAM

Step 1. Choosing the Right Aerobic Exercise Program

The following aerobic exercises will provide excellent cardiac conditioning. Other exercises, such as working the rowing machine or cross-country skiing, can be adapted by applying the same principles. Remember to avoid isometric exercises.

1. walking
2. jogging
3. stationary cycling
4. swimming
5. jump rope
6. trampoline

The following information must be determined before choosing your form of exercise.

PHYSICAL FITNESS LEVEL

If you have bad knees or ankles, walk or swim or try mild trampoline jumping. If you have been inactive, start with walking or swimming, and over several weeks slowly work up to more vigorous exercises. The walk test will help you decide where to begin. If you are able to comfortably walk 3 miles in 45 minutes, it's okay to start jogging.

AGE

If you are over forty and have been inactive for a while, avoid strenuous exercise and start with walking, swimming, low-tension stationary cycling or low-level trampoline jumping. People over sixty should stick to walking and swimming.

WHERE TO EXERCISE, INDOORS OR OUTDOORS?

This is up to you. Indoor exercises include jumping rope, stationary cycling, trampoline jumping and rowing. If you want to exercise outdoors, then choose an indoor exercise when the weather is bad.

EXPENSE

A good stationary bicycle, trampoline or rowing machine may be expensive. But walking, jogging, jumping rope and swimming do not require any expensive equipment.

Step 2. How to Pace Yourself

YOUR TARGET ZONE

If you have been inactive for a while, you must build up slowly because it takes time to get into shape. The best way to pace yourself is by exercising within your target zone (see chart on next page.)

Your target zone is 60 percent to 75 percent of your fastest heart rate. You should aim for the lower part of this range when you first begin exercising—for the first one to two months. You can slowly work up to the upper part of the range if you wish, but you will achieve maximum conditioning if you exercise anywhere in the target zone.

HOW TO MONITOR YOUR HEART RATE

The heart rate can be monitored by counting the pulse in your neck or on your wrist. Remember, this must be taken immediately when you stop exercising, because any delay will give an incorrect lower reading. The technique is as follows:

1. When you stop exercising, quickly place the second and third fingers lightly over one of the blood vessels in your neck, as shown on the diagram. These are the carotid arteries and are located on both sides of the Adam's apple on your neck. You can either count for exactly 6 seconds and add a zero, or count for 10 seconds and multiply by 6, whichever is easiest for you. For example, if you count 12 beats in 6 seconds, adding a zero gives a heart rate of 120 beats per minute; if you count 20 beats in 10 seconds, multiplying by 6 gives a heart rate of 120.

How to Find Your Target Zone

Age	Average Maximum Heart Rate (Beats per Minute)	Target Zone 60–75% (Beats per Minute)	Age	Average Maximum Heart Rate (Beats per Minute)	Target Zone 60–75% (Beats per Minute)
20	200	120–150	46	174	104–130
21	199	119–149	47	173	104–130
22	198	119–148	48	172	103–129
23	197	118–148	49	171	102–128
24	196	117–147	50	170	102–127
25	195	117–146	51	169	101–127
26	194	116–145	52	168	101–126
27	193	116–145	53	167	100–125
28	192	115–144	54	166	99–124
29	191	114–143	55	165	99–123
30	190	114–142	56	164	98–123
31	189	113–142	57	163	98–122
32	188	112–141	58	162	97–121
33	187	112–140	59	161	96–121
34	186	111–139	60	160	96–120
35	185	111–138	61	159	95–119
36	184	110–138	62	158	95–118
37	183	110–137	63	157	94–118
38	182	109–136	64	156	93–117
39	181	108–136	65	155	93–116
40	180	108–135	66	154	92–115
41	179	107–134	67	153	92–115
42	178	107–133	68	152	91–114
43	177	106–133	69	151	90–113
44	176	105–132	70	150	90–113
45	175	105–131	71	149	89–112

2. An alternate pulse location is on the inside of your wrist just below the base of your thumb, as shown on the diagram. This is the radial artery. Gently press two fingers into the groove just to the outside of the hard, cordlike structure.

3. If your pulse rate is lower than your target zone, you must exercise a little harder unless you are already tired, short of breath, or feel pain. If your pulse rate is above your target zone, you must exercise a little easier. At the beginning stop every few minutes to check your pulse to determine if you are exercising within your target zone. Then check your pulse once a week for the first three months.

Small heart rate monitors are available that attach to your earlobe, finger or chest and afford a digital readout. However, these are expensive, costing over $100 for an accurate one.

HOW LONG SHOULD YOU EXERCISE?

Every session should last for between twenty-five and forty minutes, depending on your type of exercise. This includes a five-minute warm-up period to raise the body's deep muscle temperature and to stretch the muscles and connective tissue. This prepares the body for vigorous work. It also includes a five-minute cool-down period to relax.

warm-up period	5 minutes
exercise (within target zone)	15 to 30 minutes
cool-down period	5 minutes
total	25 minutes

Step 3. The Warm-up Period

GENERAL INSTRUCTIONS

Always begin your warm-up exercise slowly, and gradually increase the pace over a five-minute period. I have included two groups of warm-up exercises here. The first set must be done for five minutes prior to the walking and the low-gear swimming exercises. The second set must be used with the jogging, jumping rope, stationary cycling, high-gear swimming, trampoline jumping and rowing exercises. They will stretch the muscles and prepare the joints you use in these vigorous activities.

GROUP 1—EXERCISE

Stretcher   Stand facing wall arms' length away. Lean forward and place palms of hands flat against wall, slightly below shoulder height. Keep back straight, heels firmly on floor, and slowly bend elbows until forehead touches wall. Tuck hips toward wall and hold position for 20 seconds. *Repeat exercise with knees slightly flexed.*

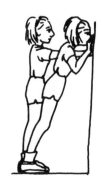

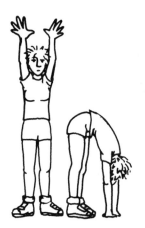

Reach and Bend   Stand erect with feet shoulder-width apart and arms extended over head. Reach as high as possible while keeping heels on floor and hold for 10 counts. Flex knees slightly and bend slowly at waist, touching floor between feet with fingers. Hold for 10 counts. (If you can't touch the floor, try to touch the tops of your shoes.) *Repeat entire sequence 2 to 5 times.*

Knee Pull   Lie flat on back with legs extended and arms at sides. Lock arms around legs just below knees and pull knees to chest, raising buttocks slightly off floor. Hold for 10 to 15 counts. (If you have knee problems, you may find it easier to lock arms behind knees.) *Repeat exercise 3 to 5 times.*

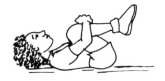

Sit-up Several versions of the sit-up are listed in reverse order of difficulty (easiest one listed first, most difficult one last). Start with the sit-up that you can do three times without undue strain. When you are able to do 10 repetitions of the exercise without great difficulty, move on to a more difficult version.

1. Lie flat on back with arms at sides, palms down, and knees slightly bent. Curl head forward until you can see past feet, hold for three counts, then lower to start position. *Repeat exercise 3 to 10 times.*

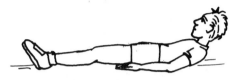

2. Lie flat on back with arms at sides, palms down, and knees slightly bent. Roll forward until upper body is at 45-degree angle to floor, then return to starting position. *Repeat exercise 3 to 10 times.*

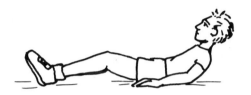

3. Lie flat on back with arms at sides, palms down, and knees slightly bent. Roll forward to sitting position, then return to starting position. *Repeat exercise 3 to 10 times.*

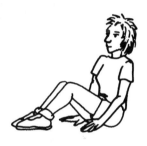

4. Lie flat on back with arms crossed on chest and knees slightly bent. Roll forward to a sitting position, then return to starting position. *Repeat exercise 3 to 10 times.*

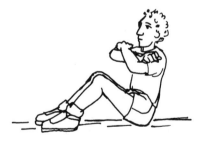

5. Lie flat on back with hands laced in back of head and knees slightly bent. Roll forward to sitting position, then return to starting position. *Repeat exercise 3 to 15 times.*

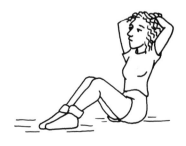

Group Two Warm-Up/Cool-Down Exercises

To minimize the chances of injury or soreness, the following exercises should be done **before** and **after** running. If you find the exercises difficult to perform, you may want to do them twice when warming up to increase flexibility. Stretch slowly and do not bounce to attain prescribed positions.

Achilles Tendon and Calf Stretcher
Stand facing wall approximately three feet away. Lean forward and place palms of hands flat against wall. Keep back straight, heels firmly on floor, and slowly bend elbows to hands, and tuck hips toward wall. Hold position for 30 seconds. *Repeat exercise with knees slightly flexed.*

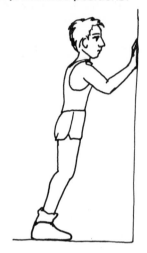

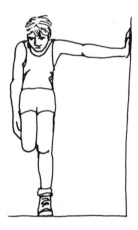

Thigh Stretcher   Stand arm's length from wall with left side toward wall. Place left hand on wall for support. Grasp right ankle with right hand and pull foot back and up until heel touches buttocks. Lean forward from waist as you lift. Hold for 30 seconds. *Repeat exercise with opposite hand and foot.*

Back Stretcher   Lie on back with legs straight and arms at sides with palms down. Slowly lift legs, hips, and lower part of back and attempt to touch toes to floor behind head. Keep legs straight and hold position for 30 seconds.

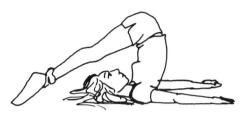

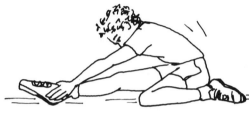

Hurdler's Stretch   Sit on floor with one leg extended straight ahead. Upper part of other leg should be at right angle to body, with heel close to buttocks. Slowly slide hands down extended leg and touch foot. Hold position for 30 seconds. Keeping legs in same position, slowly lean back and rest elbows on floor. Hold for 30 seconds. *Reverse position and repeat both stages of exercise.*

Straddle Stretch   Sit on floor and spread legs straight about twice shoulder width. Slowly lean forward from waist, sliding hands along floor, as far forward as you can. Hold for 30 seconds.

Return to starting position. Slowly stretch forward over right leg, sliding both hands down to right ankle. Try to keep knee straight and touch chin to right kneecap. Hold for 30 seconds. Return to starting position. *Repeat second step of exercise to left side.*

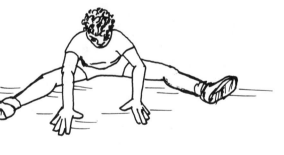

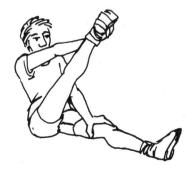

Leg Stretcher   Sit in same position as in preceding exercise. Rest left hand on left thigh and grasp inside of right foot with right hand. Keep back straight and slowly straighten right leg, letting it rise to about a 45-degree angle. Hold position for 30 seconds. *Repeat exercise with other leg.*

Your Exercise Goal

Try to exercise for a minimum of fifteen to thirty minutes each day, depending on the type of exercise you select and the intensity with which you perform it. Jogging, for example, uses more energy than walking over the same period, so jogging will take less time than walking to achieve the same conditioning effect. More vigorous exercises, such as jogging, high-gear swimming, stationary bicycling and trampoline jumping, only have to be performed for at least fifteen minutes. But walking and mild swimming should be done for a minimum of thirty minutes. All the exercise programs require that you build up slowly over several weeks.

AEROBIC EXERCISE PROGRAMS

The 14-Day Walking Program

Walking is an excellent cardiac conditioning program. Besides, you don't have to take lessons to learn how to walk, almost everyone can do it, it doesn't cost anything, it is virtually injury free and has the lowest dropout rate of any form of exercise. Walking has recently gained new respect as a means of improving physical fitness if it is performed at a brisk pace for at least fifteen to twenty minutes in a rhythmic fashion. Moreover, it is an excellent aerobic exercise for older individuals and people with knee injuries and other medical problems that preclude jogging.

Walk briskly at a steady clip. Don't saunter, stroll or shuffle. The object is to walk fast enough to get your pulse up into your target zone. Follow these tips.

1. Hold your head erect and keep your back straight and your abdomen flat.
2. Point your toes straight ahead and swing your arms loosely at your sides.
3. Land on the heel of the foot and roll forward to drive off the ball of the foot. Walking only on the ball of the foot or in a flat-footed style may cause fatigue and soreness.
4. Take long, easy strides but don't strain for distance.
5. Lean forward slightly when walking up or down hills or at a very rapid pace.
6. Breathe deeply, with your mouth open if that is more comfortable.
7. At the beginning of the program, stop suddenly every five minutes and immediately take your pulse. If it is lower than the lowest part of

your target zone, you must speed up. If it is faster than the upper part of your target zone, slow down your pace. After you get your pace up to your target zone for a few days, then you can check your pulse twice a week.

DAYS 1–5

5 minutes	group 1 warm-up cool-down exercises
5 minutes	brisk walk
5 minutes	group 1 warm-up cool-down exercises

DAYS 6–10

5 minutes	group 1 warm-up cool-down exercises
7 minutes	brisk walk
5 minutes	group 1 warm-up cool-down exercises

DAYS 11–14

5 minutes	group 1 warm-up cool-down exercises
9 minutes	brisk walk
5 minutes	group 1 warm-up cool-down exercises

The 14-Day Jogging Program

Since jogging is a very strenuous exercise, start with brisk walking and gradually increase the running phase by about two minutes each week. When you first begin running, progress will appear slow, but gradually in the weeks ahead you will become aware that your strength and staying power are increasing. It is important to understand that the time you spend jogging is more important than the speed of jogging.

Heed the following suggestions before beginning to jog:

1. The right pace can be determined by taking the *talk test*. You should be able to talk while alternately running and walking. If you are too breathless to talk, you are going too fast.
2. Run in an upright position, avoiding excessive forward lean. Keep your back as straight as you comfortably can and keep your head up. Do not look at your feet. (See diagram on page 31.)

3. Carry your arms away from the body, with elbows bent so that your forearms are roughly parallel to the ground.
4. Shake out and relax your arms occasionally to prevent shoulder tightness.
5. Land on the heel of the foot and rock forward to drive off the ball of the foot. If this proves to be difficult, try a more flat-footed style. Running on the balls of your feet will tire you quickly and make the legs sore.
6. Keep your stride relatively short. Don't force your pace by reaching for extra distance.
7. Breathe deeply, with your mouth open.
8. Wear the proper clothes for the weather.

If you can pass the *walk test* by comfortably walking 3 miles in 45 minutes, you can bypass the first fourteen days and begin this program with weeks 4 and 5 in chapter 10. If you can't pass the test, you must start at the beginning of this program (Days 1–5). If you find you are tired or breathless at any stage of the program, either work on the previous week's schedule or modify it to build up less quickly.

DAYS 1–5

5 minutes	group 2 warm-up cool-down exercises
10 minutes	brisk walk, preferably without stopping
3 minutes	walk slowly
2 minutes	group 2 warm-up cool-down exercises

DAYS 6–10

5 minutes	group 2 warm-up cool-down exercises
5 minutes	brisk walk, preferably without stopping
1 minute	jog
5 minutes	brisk walk
1 minute	jog
3 minutes	walk slowly
2 minutes	group 2 warm-up cool-down exercises

Good and Bad Running Form

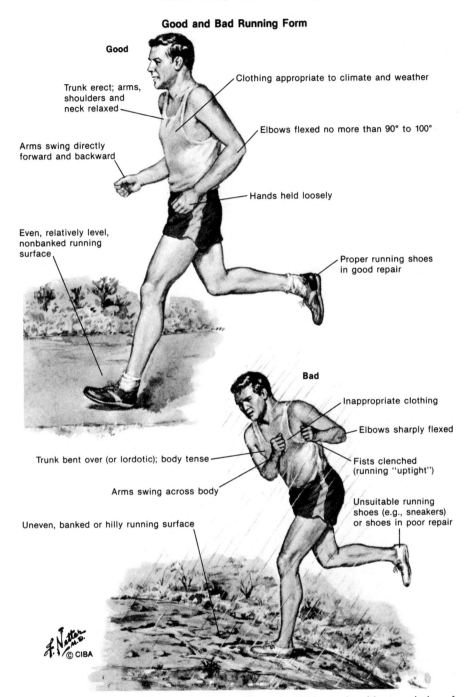

Good

Trunk erect; arms, shoulders and neck relaxed

Clothing appropriate to climate and weather

Elbows flexed no more than 90° to 100°

Arms swing directly forward and backward

Hands held loosely

Even, relatively level, nonbanked running surface

Proper running shoes in good repair

Bad

Inappropriate clothing

Elbows sharply flexed

Trunk bent over (or lordotic); body tense

Fists clenched (running "uptight")

Arms swing across body

Unsuitable running shoes (e.g., sneakers) or shoes in poor repair

Uneven, banked or hilly running surface

Illustration by Frank Netter from *Clinical Symposia*, 1980, reprinted by permission of Ciba Pharmaceutical Co.

DAYS 11—14

5 minutes	group 2 warm-up cool-down exercises
5 minutes	brisk walk
2 minutes	jog
5 minutes	brisk walk
2 minutes	jog
3 minutes	walk slowly
2 minutes	group 2 warm-up cool-down exercises

The 14-Day Stationary Cycling Program

Stationary cycling is one of the easiest of the aerobic exercises to maintain your pulse in the target zone. This program requires a cycle with a tension device that can be adjusted to increase the work load by applying resistance to pedaling.

Remember the following points in getting started:

1. Adjust the seat so your body is bent slightly forward and your knees have a slight bend when your feet on the pedals are in the down position and your hands are on the handle grips (Fig. 2.1). The

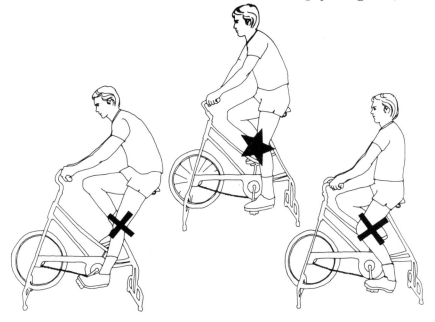

The Correct Seat Height for Bicycling.
With toe on pedal, there should be a small bend at the knee.

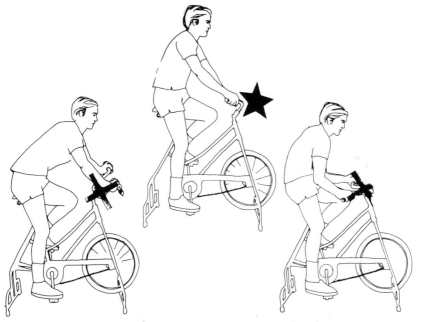

The Correct Handlebar Position for Bicycling.
The body should be relaxed and leaning slightly forward.

optimum seat-to-pedal distance is 2 inches added to the person's crotch-to-floor measurement.

2. Direct the handlebar toward the cyclist with a slight tilt upward. Never direct the handlebar toward the front of the cycle or downward (Fig. 2.2).

3. The resistance control adjustment device is used to increase the work load (Fig. 2.3). Maintain a constant cycling rate and adjust the device gradually according to your pulse rate. In practice, begin cycling in the range of 40 to 60 cycles a minute and then stop abruptly to take your pulse. If it is below your target zone, slowly adjust the tension, cycle at the same rate and take your pulse again. Repeat this until you are in your target zone. The resistance control devices on the more expensive cycles such as Monarch and Tunturi are very accurate and allow you to use the same setting reproducibly from day to day. Once the resistance device is set to your target zone, you will be able to use this setting anytime you exercise. But on the inexpensive cycles, the resistance device is not very accurate and is rarely calibrated. You can still use some of these bikes, however, by marking the knob and counting turns.

You should always check the knob before buying a bike, because

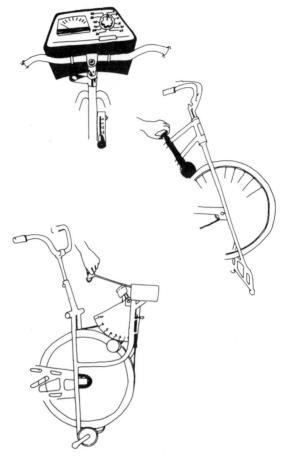

Various Types of Bicycle Resistance Controls. a. Stationary bicycle where resistance is altered electronically in proportion to the pedaling speed. Resistance level is constant and reproducible. b. Friction braked bicycles have a knob which applies resistance that is difficult to reproduce. c. Mechanically braked bicycles are braked by a weighted belt running around the rim. Resistance level is reproducible.

some are too hard to grip or turn. The Schwinn Deluxe cycle is relatively inexpensive, and although the resistance control device isn't calibrated, it can easily be adjusted. In addition the Schwinn offers other features that are superior to those in some of the more expensive bikes. If you purchase an inexpensive bike, when your pulse rate is on target, mark the resistance control. The next time you exercise you may have to adjust it slightly by checking your pulse rate. With a little practice, this will become second nature.

4. In order to eliminate boredom, place your cycle in front of the television during exercise and watch a selected program at the same time each day.

DAYS 1–5

5 minutes	group 2 warm-up cool-down exercises
5 minutes	cycle at 60 cycles a minute without tension
5 minutes	cycle at 60 cycles a minute with slight tension to your target zone
5 minutes	group 2 warm-up cool-down exercises

DAYS 6–10

5 minutes	group 2 warm-up cool-down exercises
3 minutes	cycle at 60 cycles a minute without tension
7 minutes	cycle at 60 cycles a minute with slight tension to your target zone
5 minutes	group 2 warm-up cool-down exercises

DAYS 11–14

5 minutes	group 2 warm-up cool-down exercises
2 minutes	cycle at 60 cycles a minute without tension
10 minutes	cycle at 60 cycles a minute with slight tension to your target zone
5 minutes	group 2 warm-up cool-down exercises

The 14-Day Jump Rope Program

Simple and versatile, skipping rope is an excellent exercise for cardiac conditioning. It can be done year-round regardless of inclement weather, can be packed in a suitcase when going on a trip and can be adapted to music. Conditioning can be accomplished for some individuals with slow jumping speeds, as jumping rope can raise the heart rate quite rapidly. People with ankle and knee problems should not jump rope.

There are certain requirements that must be met to make jumping rope a productive exercise program.

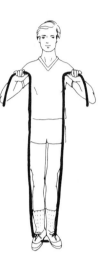

1. Adjust the jump rope by placing the center of the rope under both feet and bringing each end along the outside of the legs and up under the armpits. This is just about the right length with handles included. Cut or adjust the excess to this length.
2. Place your arms at your sides with a 35- to 45-degree bend at the elbows and your forearms several inches away from your body.
3. Using a wrist action, swing the rope with both hands in a complete arc under your feet. At the moment the rope approaches the feet, jump just enough for rope clearance and no more (about an inch).
4. Practice one jump at a time until you get the hang of it; then continue jumping in a repetitive, rhythmic motion.

DAYS 1–5

5 minutes	group 2 warm-up cool-down exercises
25 times	jump without rope, and swing arms
1 minute	take a brisk walk
25 times	jump with rope slowly
1 minute	take a brisk walk
5 minutes	group 2 warm-up cool-down exercises

DAYS 6–10

5 minutes	group 2 warm-up cool-down exercises
50 times	jump with rope slowly
2 minutes	take a brisk walk
50 times	jump rope, taking the pulse and keeping it in the lower part of the target zone
5 minutes	group 2 warm-up cool-down exercises

DAYS 11–14

5 minutes	group 2 warm-up cool-down exercises
50 times	jump rope, taking the pulse and staying in the lower part of the target zone
1 minute	take a brisk walk
50 times	jump rope, taking the pulse and staying in the lower part of the target zone
5 minutes	group 2 warm-up cool-down exercises

The 14-Day Swimming Program

Swimming is one of the best exercises for people of all ages, including the handicapped. It is a highly efficient exercise program that adapts to myriad exercise programs, is a lot of fun, rarely causes muscle or joint injuries, provides programs for older individuals and is relatively inexpensive.

Activities can be performed more easily in water because of the decrease in gravitational pull. When a person is submerged up to the neck, there is an apparent loss of about 90 percent of body weight, so that a person weighing 130 pounds only has to support a weight of 13 pounds on his or her legs and feet. This is particularly beneficial for older people with painful joints and weak muscles, as it makes it more comfortable for them to exercise. Moreover, many people who are not able to jog on land will be able to jog in the water. (An excellent conditioning activity in the high-gear exercise program is *bobbing*, in which the head and shoulders are pushed out of the water the same way a cork held underwater bobs when it is released. During bobbing activities, the demands for breathing are great.)

This program consists of two levels of exercise: low gear and high gear. It is important that you monitor your pulse and adjust your speed accordingly when performing the swimming exercises.

Most home swimming pools range from 35 to 45 feet in length. The Amateur Athletic Union (AAU) rules recommend a length of 75 feet for indoor competition and a length of about 165 feet for outdoor competition. The pool length in the following exercise programs is based on a home swimming pool. If any other size pool is used, adjust your exercise accordingly.

Toe Bounce

Standing in waist-to-chest deep
water with hands on hips,
swimmer:

(1) Jumps high with feet together through a bounding
movement of the feet.
Repeat.

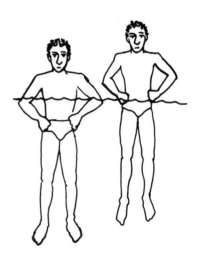

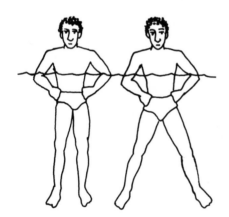

Side Straddle Hop

Standing in waist-to-chest deep
water with hands on hips,
swimmer:

(1) Jumps sideward to position
with feet approximately
two feet apart.
(2) Recovers.

Elementary Treading

In water deep enough that toes
will not touch bottom, in a per-
pendicular position, swimmer:

(1) Sculls or fins as he kicks
bicycle, scissors, or frog
style.

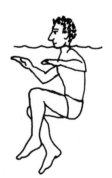

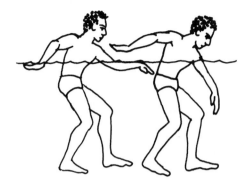

Standing Crawl

Standing in waist-to-chest deep water, swimmer:

(1) Simulates the overhand crawl stroke by.
  (a) Reaching out with the left hand, getting a grip on the water, pressing downward and pulling, bringing the left hand through to the thigh.
  (b) Reaching out with the right hand, etc. Repeat.

Front Flutter Kicking

Lying in a prone position and holding on to side of pool with hand(s), swimmer:

(1) Kicks flutter-style in which toes are pointed back, ankles are flexible, knee joint is loose but straight and the whole leg acts as a whip.

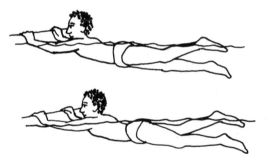

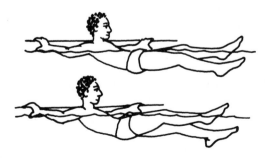

Back Flutter Kicking

Lying in a supine position and holding on to sides of pool with hand(s), swimmer:

(1) Flutter kicks.

Power Bobbing

Power bobbing is similar to "high bobbing" except that at the top of the upward thrust the hands scull vigorously as the legs flutter kick. In "power bobbing" the swimmer will literally blast out of the water exposing all of the body to the hips.

Bobbing is a well-rounded workout involving leg power, arm and shoulder work, heavy forced breathing, and rhythmical vigorous action.

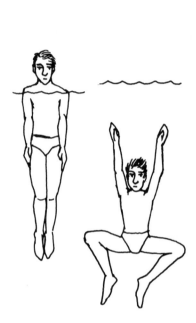

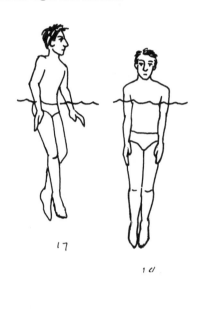

High Bobbing

In water approximately one to three feet over the swimmer's head, swimmer:

(1) Takes a vertical position, hands extended outward from the sides with palms turned downward. Legs are drawn in position for frog kick.

(2) Simultaneously pulls hands sharply to thighs with legs executing frog kick.

(3) Inhales at peak of height.

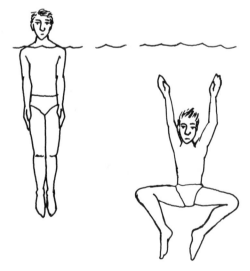

High Bobbing (cont.)

(4) Drops with thrust of arms downward with palms turned upward until feet reach bottom of the pool and tucks to a squat position. Exhales throughout this action.

(5) Jumps upward with power leg thrust at the same time pulling arms in a breast stroke position downward, causing the head and shoulders to rise high out of water. Exhales during (4) and (5).

(6) Inhales and repeats cycles (4) and (5), etc.

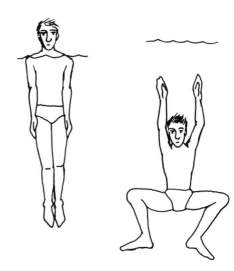

Advanced Bobbing

Treading in deep water, swimmer:

(1) Assumes a vertical position with hands extended outward from the sides, just under the surface of the water, with palms turned downward. Legs are drawn in a position of readiness for a frog or scissors kick.

(2) Executes kick as hands are pulled sharply to thighs and legs. (As a result of this action, the head and shoulders rise out of the water and a deep breath is taken at the highest point reached.)

(3) As the body sinks, the arms are outstretched overhead and swimmer exhales. Repeat (1), (2), and (3).

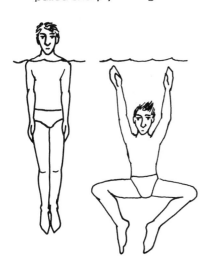

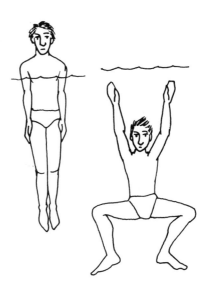

Low-Gear Exercise Program

5 minutes	group 1 warm-up cool-down exercises
15 seconds	toe bounce
30 seconds	standing crawl
15 seconds	side straddle hop
30 seconds	front flutter
30 seconds	elementary treading
as indicated for each day	lap swimming
2 minutes	group 3 warm-up cool-down exercises

DAYS 1—5

Do the low-gear exercise program as defined. The lap swimming is done by swimming one length of the pool, getting out, walking back and repeating five times. Each day increase by 1 minute the time you spend swimming laps, and monitor your pulse.

DAYS 6—10

Do the same routine except swim two lengths of the pool, get out and walk back. Repeat five times, adding one additional repetition each day. Monitor your pulse.

DAYS 11—14

Do the same routine except swim three lengths of the pool, get out and walk back. Repeat five times. Add one additional repetition on day thirteen. Monitor your pulse.

High-Gear Exercise Program

2 minutes	group 3 warm-up cool-down exercises
3 minutes	front flutter
3 minutes	back flutter
3 minutes	advanced bobbing
3 minutes	high bobbing
1 minute	power bobbing
as indicated	lap swimming
2 minutes	group 3 warm-up cool-down exercises

DAYS 1–5

Do the high-gear exercises as indicated. The lap swimming should be done by swimming three lengths of the pool, getting out, walking back and repeating three times. Add one additional repetition each day. Monitor your pulse.

DAYS 6–10

The same as for days 1 to 5, except do four lengths of the pool and repeat three times. Add one additional repetition on day 8 and another on day 10. Monitor your pulse.

DAYS 11–14

The same as for days 6 to 10, except do five lengths of the pool and repeat three times. Add one additional repetition on day 13. Monitor your pulse.

The 14-Day Trampoline Program

Trampoline exercises on a shock-absorbing type of trampoline provide an interesting, highly efficient form of cardiac conditioning. Trampolines measure 7 inches from the floor and are 36 to 46 inches square (or in diameter). The shock-absorbing action makes it attractive to anyone with a knee, ankle or back problem, since it reduces trauma to these areas. Many types of procedures can easily be adapted to this form of exercise, making it a lot of fun. One good series of trampoline exercises, called the rotating program, consists of running in place 40 times, rotating another 90 degrees, doing jumping jacks (butterflies) 30 times, rotating 90 degrees, then doing back kicks 30 times, rotating 90 degrees, then doing body twists 30 times. Repeat these continuously for 20 minutes. Instead of this rotating sequence, beneficial effects can be accomplished by performing any single exercise, such as running in place, jumping jack, fast walk, and so on.

Walking-Type Program on the Trampoline, Day 1–Day 14

1. Do 5 minutes of the group 1 warm-up cool-down exercises.
2. Stand on the mat with your feet apart.
3. A walking-type program is done by bending one knee and lifting the heel. Then do the same with the other leg while swinging the arms rhythmically back and forth.
4. Do a modification of the 14-Day Walking Program, with careful monitoring of your pulse within your target zone.
5. Do 5 minutes of the group 1 warm-up cool-down exercises.

Jogging-Type Program on the Trampoline, Day 1–Day 14

1. Do 5 minutes of the group 2 warm-up cool-down exercises.
2. Stand on the mat with your feet apart and begin to lift each leg slightly off the mat in a jogging motion, developing a running type of rhythm.
3. This exercise is made more strenuous by increasing the height of the knee, and the running speed.
4. Use a modification of the 14-Day Jogging Program on page 29 and the 14-Day Walking Program on page 28, with careful monitoring of your pulse to maintain your rate within your target zone.
5. Do 5 minutes of the group 2 warm-up cool-down exercises.

Mixed Routine, Day 1–Day 14

This combination of several rotating exercises should be used only after three to four weeks of conditioning at a lower activity level. The four exercises in the following routine are running in place, then doing jumping jacks (butterflies), back kicks and body twists.

1. Do 5 minutes of the group 2 warm-up cool-down exercises.
2. Run in place 40 times.
3. Rotate 90 degrees clockwise.
4. Do the jumping jack (butterfly) 30 times.
5. Rotate another 90 degrees clockwise.
6. Run by stooping forward and kicking each foot backward in sequence.
7. Rotate another 90 degrees clockwise.
8. Place your hands on your hips and twist the torso by turning the body at the waist from left to right, 25 times.
9. Do this exercise continuously for 20 minutes, with careful monitoring of your pulse to be certain you don't exceed your target range.
10. Slow down for about 2 minutes.
11. Do 3 minutes of the group 2 warm-up cool-down exercises.

Modify this program by substituting or adding to it any exercise you wish. Try doing it to music, as in aerobic dancing.

EXERCISE ATTIRE

If your choice of exercise is jogging or walking, a well-made pair of jogging shoes is indispensable to prevent injuries. They should have heavy cushioned soles, provide good support, contain arch supports and be comfortable. The specifications of a good running shoe are provided in the following illustration.

Always listen to the dictates of the weather. Since jogging and fast walking generate a lot of heat, you must wear lighter clothing when it is warm, and never wear plastic or rubber clothing that prevents evaporation and may cause the body temperature to rise to dangerous levels. A rule of thumb is to use light shades of clothing and a white hat in the summer to reflect the rays of the sun, and dark shades in the winter to absorb the heat. But remember to wear a reflector of some sort in the evening so that passing automobiles see you. Dress warmly in the winter by wearing several layers of light clothing rather than one or two heavy layers, since the extra layers trap heat and it's easy to shed one of the layers if it becomes too warm. If you are properly dressed, you can jog in almost any weather. On hot, humid days, exercise when it is cooler—in the early morning or after sundown.

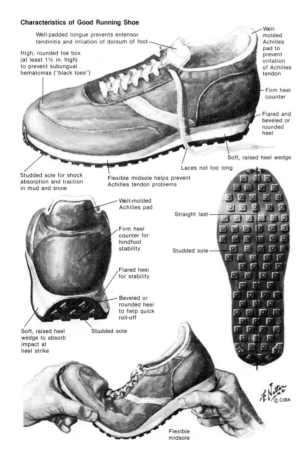

Characteristics of Good Running Shoe

Well-padded tongue prevents extensor tendinitis and irritation of dorsum of foot

High, rounded toe box (at least 1½ in. high) to prevent subungual hematomas ("black toes")

Well-molded Achilles pad to prevent irritation of Achilles tendon

Firm heel counter

Flared and beveled or rounded heel

Soft, raised heel wedge

Laces not too long

Studded sole for shock absorption and traction in mud and snow

Flexible midsole helps prevent Achilles tendon problems

Well-molded Achilles pad

Straight last

Firm heel counter for hindfoot stability

Studded sole

Flared heel for stability

Beveled or rounded heel to help quick roll-off

Soft, raised heel wedge to absorb impact at heel strike

Studded sole

Flexible midsole

Illustration by Frank Netter from *Clinical Symposia*, 1980, reprinted by permission of Ciba Pharmaceutical Co.

KEEPING ACTIVE

Don't restrict physical activity to your exercise program but make it a way of life. Whenever opportunities arise to be physically active, take advantage of them.

1. Use the stairs instead of the elevator. Start with one flight and gradually increase the number.
2. Walk to work if you live at a reasonable distance.
3. Park a few blocks from work and walk the remaining distance.
4. If you use public transportation, get off one or two stops before your regular one and walk.
5. Take a stroll during coffee breaks.

HOW TO AVOID INJURIES AND SERIOUS ILLNESS

Danger Signals

Cardiac Problems

If you experience any of the following symptoms while exercising, *stop your exercise and call your doctor immediately.* Ignoring these signals and continuing to exercise may lead to serious consequences.

1. sudden onset of pain in the chest, arm, neck, shoulder or jaw
2. sudden onset of shortness of breath
3. sudden onset of cold sweats
4. sudden onset of dizziness
5. sudden onset of pallor
6. sudden onset of fainting

ATHLETIC INJURIES

Excessive exercise; improper shoes; running on uneven surfaces and concrete sidewalks, up and down curbs; uphill running; downhill running; and bad running form can cause injuries to the joints, feet, ankles and legs. Listen to your body when you exercise and pay heed to early warning pains in these areas. Don't compete with others until you become experienced and well conditioned.

OTHER PROBLEMS

Engaging in outdoor exercises such as jogging can predispose a person to heat injuries such as heat cramps, heat exhaustion and heat stroke. During exercise the body regulates its temperature through sweating. But if over-sweating occurs, any of these heat injuries can occur, depending on how much you sweat.

YOUR EXERCISE PRESCRIPTION FOR A HEALTHY HEART

Make a lifelong commitment to incorporating the 14-Day Heart-Saving Exercise Plan into your daily schedule so that it becomes an integral part of your life-style. In this way you will be exercising your way to a healthy heart.

Chapter Three

The 14-Day Heart-Saving

Diet Plan

All human history attests
That happiness for man—the hungry sinner!—
Since Eve ate apples, much depends on dinner.
—Lord Byron

The 14-Day Heart-Saving Diet Plan will change your eating habits so that your total cholesterol, bad cholesterol and triglyceride levels will decrease, your good cholesterol will increase and your high blood pressure will become lower.

Adhering to a low-fat, low-cholesterol diet requires making a drastic change in your eating habits. Make this change gradually. A sudden shift in diet leads to failure even when it is made for serious medical reasons.

Begin losing weight if you have an elevated triglyceride level, are diabetic or are more than 20 percent overweight. (See the height and weight tables in Appendix B, which indicate the weights at which mortality is lowest and longevity is highest.) Actually any person who is overweight, regardless of the amount, should reduce. Any successful diet to reduce elevated triglycerides in your blood requires weight reduction as the single most important step. The blood triglyceride levels usually drop very quickly after weight reduction and generally stay down as long as the person's weight remains in the normal range. Weight reduction also commonly reverses the diabetic state and lowers high blood pressure. (Diabetics who are on insulin or oral agents should always lose weight under the supervision of their physicians.) Another important health benefit of this diet relates to your increase of daily fiber intake (plant fibers that pass through the intestine without being digested).

Health Benefits of a High-Fiber Diet

Fewer heart attacks occur among people on high-fiber diets. Such people also show a reduction in blood cholesterol and triglyceride levels. No one knows whether this is due to a binding effect by the fiber or in part to a lower fat and cholesterol intake at the expense of the higher fiber intake.

Colon cancer, diabetes, hemorrhoids, appendicitis, hiatus hernia, diverticulosis (pockets in the colon) and other diseases also occur less among people with high-fiber diets. For example, colon cancer, which results in the second highest number of cancer deaths in the United States, is rare among certain Africans who eat high-fiber diets consisting of bananas and millet seeds. Those African natives who took on Western habits, however, had an incidence rate similar to the Americans. Perhaps people on low-fiber diets keep bacteria in contact with the wall of the colon for prolonged periods of time, giving toxins time to cause the cancer. Diabetes was also rare in African tribes eating high-fiber diets.

There are two major groups of fiber that are important to nutrition: *soluble* fibers and *insoluble* fibers. Soluble fibers are used by plants for repair purposes. They include the gelatinous substance *pectin*, and the gumlike substance *guar*. Pectin is a carbohydrate found in most fruits and vegetables, especially apples, plums, blackberries, carrots, beans, cranberries and crabapples. It is used to stiffen or thicken food substances like jellies. Guar is extracted from the cluster bean and other bean products or from the seeds or stems of tropical plants. Soluble fibers have a slower transit time in leaving the stomach and passing through the intestines. They bind various substances in the intestines, such as sugars and perhaps cholesterol and certain fats, resulting in lower blood levels of these substances.

Insoluble fibers, however, are essentially untouched by the enzymes in the digestive tract. They include cellulose, hemicellulose and lignin—all parts of the cell wall of plants. Bran, grain cereals and whole-grain breads are the key members of this group. They have the capacity to absorb large amounts of water, thereby causing a bulkier stool, which promotes rapid and easier passage through the intestines. This rapid passage may also interfere with sugar, fat and cholesterol absorption.

Before starting the 14-Day Heart-Saving Diet Plan, let's review the principles of this eating program.

The formula for changing your body chemistry is this:

1. You need not cut the total amount of food you eat so long as the diet is properly balanced, you are not overweight and you are maintaining a desirable body weight (see table in Appendix B).

2. The total number of calories you get from the fat in your food must not exceed 30% of the total calories you consume from all sources— fats, proteins and carbohydrates combined.
3. The total calories coming from the fat you eat must be distributed as follows:

   • The saturated fat intake in your food must be less than 10% of the total number of all the calories you consume.
   • The polyunsaturated fat intake in your food should be in the vicinity of but should not exceed 10% of the total calories that you consume.

4. The daily cholesterol intake should be less than 250 milligrams.
5. Complex carbohydrates (vegetables, beans, nuts, some fruits, grains, etc.) should constitute at least 50% to 60% of the total calories you eat. The sucrose intake must be markedly reduced.
6. A high-fiber diet must be instituted at the same time. This will increase the complex carbohydrate intake and provide for a lower fat and cholesterol intake.
7. Dietary supplements may be used as recommended in chapter 7 (vitamins A, B_6, C and E, magnesium, chromium and selenium).

THE 14-DAY HEART-SAVING MENU PLAN

If you are overweight, let's begin the 14-Day Heart-Saving Program by losing weight! First, refer to the Low-Fat Low-Cholesterol Weight Reduction Plan in Appendix A to determine your calorie level to lose at least 2 pounds each week.

The following 1200-calorie low-fat, low-cholesterol diet plan serves as an example of a two-week menu program that incorporates an exchange technique that is easy to use, adds variety to your meals and at the same time will lower your total cholesterol, bad cholesterol and triglycerides and raise your good cholesterol. Consult the Food Exchange chart in Appendix B to make any changes in the menus according to your liking.

Day 1: 1200 Calories

Meal	Food	Exchange
Breakfast	1 cup grapefruit juice	2 fruit
	2 slices whole wheat toast	2 bread
	1 tsp. margarine	1 fat
	1 cup black coffee or tea	free

| Mid-A.M. | 1 cup chicken broth | free |
| Snack | 1 cup black coffee or tea | free |

Lunch	1 cup lettuce, for salad	2 vegetable
	1½ oz. cold cuts, diced	½ meat
	1 tbsp. Italian dressing	1 fat
	1 peach	1 fruit
	1 cup black coffee or tea	free

| Mid-P.M. | 1 apple | 1 fruit |
| Snack | 1 cup black coffee or tea | free |

Dinner	3 oz. turkey	1 meat
	½ cup mashed potatoes	1 bread
	2 tbsp. meatless fat-free gravy	free
	½ cup peas	1 vegetable
	½ cup carrots	1 vegetable
	1 tsp. margarine	1 fat
	½ cup sherbet	3 fruit
		.2 fat
	1 cup black coffee or tea	free

Evening	1 cup broth	free
Snack	1 cup skim milk	1 milk
	1 cup coffee or tea	free

Day 2: 1200 Calories

Meal	Food	Exchange
Breakfast	1 cup orange juice	2 fruit
	2 English muffin halves	2 bread
	1 tsp. margarine	1 fat
	1 cup black coffee or tea	free

| Mid-A.M. | 2 plums | 1 fruit |
| Snack | 1 cup black coffee or tea | free |

Lunch	1 cup fruit cocktail	2 fruit
	½ cup carrot sticks	1 vegetable
	1 cup black coffee or tea	free

| Mid-P.M. Snack | 1 graham cracker | 1 bread |
| | 1 cup black coffee or tea | free |

Dinner	4½ oz. chicken	1.5 meat
	1 cup rice	2 bread
	2 tbsp. meatless fat-free gravy	free
	1 cup lettuce, for salad	2 vegetable
	½ cup tomatoes	1 vegetable
	⅓ cup Jell-O	1 bread
	½ cup blueberries	1 fruit
	1 cup black coffee or tea	free

Evening Snack	1 peach	1 fruit
	1 cup skim milk	1 milk
	1 cup coffee or tea	free

Day 3: 1200 Calories

Meal	**Food**	**Exchange**
Breakfast	1 cup orange juice	2 fruit
	1 bagel	2 bread
	1 tsp. margarine	1 fat
	1 cup black coffee or tea	free
Mid-A.M. Snack	1 apple	1 fruit
	1 cup black coffee or tea	free
Lunch	10 oz. green pea soup	1 vegetable
	3 soda crackers	1 bread
	1 cup black coffee or tea	free
Mid-P.M. Snack	2 marshmallows	1 fruit
	1 cup black coffee or tea	free
Dinner	4½ oz. steak	1.5 meat
	1 baked potato	1 bread
	1 tsp. margarine	1 fat
	½ cup lettuce, for salad	1 vegetable
	½ cup carrots	1 vegetable
	1 tsp. margarine	1 fat

	½ cup applesauce	1 fruit
	½ cup fruit cocktail	1 fruit
	1 cup black coffee or tea	free
Evening Snack	1 peach	1 fruit
	1 cup skim milk	1 milk
	1 cup coffee or tea	free

Day 4: 1200 Calories

Meal	Food	Exchange
Breakfast	⅔ cup apple juice	2 fruit
	½ cup dry cereal	2 bread
	½ cup skim milk	.5 milk
	1 cup black coffee or tea	free
Mid-A.M. Snack	½ bagel	1 bread
	1 tsp. margarine	1 fat
	1 cup black coffee or tea	free
Lunch	1 cup lettuce, for salad	2 vegetable
	1 tbsp. French dressing	1 fat
	1 apple	1 fruit
	1 cup black coffee or tea	free
Mid-P.M. Snack	1 pear	1 fruit
	1 cup black coffee or tea	free
Dinner	4½ oz. chicken in lemon	1.5 meat
	1 cup rice	1 bread
	1 tsp. margarine	1 fat
	½ cup peas	1 vegetable
	½ cup cranberry sauce	1 fruit
	½ cup spinach	1 vegetable
	1 cup black coffee or tea	free
Evening Snack	½ cup fruit cocktail	1 fruit
	½ cup skim milk	1 milk
	1 cup coffee or tea	free

Day 5: 1200 Calories

Meal	Food	Exchange
Breakfast	1 cup orange juice	2 fruit
	1 hard roll, small	1 bread
	1 tsp. margarine	1 fat
	1 cup black coffee or tea	free
Mid-A.M. Snack	½ bagel	1 bread
	1 tsp. margarine	1 fat
	1 cup black coffee or tea	free
Lunch	10 oz. tomato soup	1 vegetable
	3 soda crackers	1 bread
	2 plums	1 fruit
	1 cup black coffee or tea	free
Mid-P.M. Snack	1 peach	1 fruit
	1 cup black coffee or tea	free
Dinner	4½ oz. fish fillet	1.5 meat
	1 cup rice	1 bread
	1 tsp. margarine	fat
	1 cup mixed vegetables	1 vegetable
	½ cup lettuce for salad	1 vegetable
	1 tbsp. Italian dressing	1 fat
	1 cup black coffee or tea	free
Evening Snack	½ cup fruit cocktail	1 fruit
	1 cup skim milk	1 milk
	1 cup coffee or tea	free

Day 6: 1200 Calories

Meal	Food	Exchange
Breakfast	1 cup orange juice	2 fruit
	1 cup hot cereal	2 bread
	½ cup skim milk	.5 milk
	1 cup black coffee or tea	free

| Mid-A.M. Snack | ½ cup grapefruit | 1 fruit |
| | 1 cup black coffee or tea | free |

Lunch	1 peanut butter sandwich	2 bread
	2 tsp. peanut butter	2 fat
	2 plums	1 fruit
	1 cup black coffee or tea, or	free
	1 bottle sugar-free beverage	free

| Mid-P.M. Snack | ½ cup carrot sticks | 1 vegetable |
| | 1 cup coffee or tea | free |

Dinner	4½ oz. lamb	1½ meat
	½ cup mashed potatoes	1 bread
	½ cup asparagus	1 vegetable
	lettuce, for salad	1 vegetable
	(no restriction on amount)	
	1 tbsp. French dressing	1 fat
	½ cup applesauce	1 fruit
	1 3-inch cube angel-food cake	1 bread
	1 cup black coffee or tea	free

| Evening Snack | ½ cup skim milk | .5 milk |
| | 1 orange | 1 fruit |

Day 7: 1200 Calories

Meal	**Food**	**Exchange**
Breakfast	1 cup orange juice	2 fruit
	1 English muffin	2 bread
	1 tsp. margarine	1 fat
	1 cup black coffee or tea	free
Mid-A.M. Snack	1 apple	1 fruit
	1 cup black coffee or tea	free
Lunch	10 oz. chicken gumbo soup	1 vegetable
	1 slice whole-wheat bread	1 bread
	1 tsp. margarine	1 fat
	1 cup black coffee or tea or	free
	1 bottle sugar-free beverage	free

Mid-P.M. Snack	¾ cup low-fat yogurt 1 cup black coffee or tea	1 milk free
Dinner	4½ oz. turkey ½ cup macaroni 1 tsp. fat-free gravy ½ cup tomatoes ½ cup broccoli ½ cup Jell-O 1 cup strawberries 1 cup black coffee or tea	1½ meat 1 bread 1 free 1 vegetable 1 vegetable 1 bread 1 fruit free
Evening Snack	1 cup coffee or tea 1 banana	free 2 fruit

Day 8: 1200 Calories

Meal	**Food**	**Exchange**
Breakfast	1 cup orange juice 1 cup hot cereal ½ cup skim milk 1 cup black coffee or tea	2 fruit 2 bread .5 milk free
Mid-A.M. Snack	1 banana 1 cup black coffee or tea	2 fruit free
Lunch	½ cup lettuce, for salad 1 tbsp. French dressing ½ cup fruit cocktail 1 cup black coffee, tea or 1 bottle sugar-free beverage	1 vegetable 1 fat 1 fruit free free
Mid-P.M. Snack	½ grapefruit 1 cup black coffee or tea	1 fruit free
Dinner	4½ oz. pork chop 1 cup rice 1 tbsp. fat-free gravy ½ cup Brussels sprouts	1½ meat 2 bread 1 free 1 vegetable

	½ cup mushrooms	1 vegetable
	1½-inch cube angel-food cake	1 bread
	1 cup black coffee or tea	free
Evening	1 cup coffee or tea	free
Snack	1 tangerine	1 fruit

Day 9: 1200 Calories

Meal	Food	Exchange
Breakfast	⅔ cup apple juice	2 fruit
	1½ cup dry cereal	2 bread
	½ cup skim milk	.5 milk
	1 cup black coffee or tea	free
Mid-A.M.	2 plums	1 fruit
Snack	1 cup black coffee or tea	free
Lunch	10 oz. vegetable beef soup	1 vegetable
	1 slice white bread	1 bread
	1 tsp. margarine	1 fat
	1 cup black coffee or tea or	free
	1 bottle sugar-free beverage	free
Mid-P.M.	¼ cantaloupe	1 fruit
Snack	1 cup black coffee or tea	free
Dinner	1 cup spaghetti	2 bread
	½ cup tomato sauce	1 vegetable
	4½ oz. lean ground beef	1.5 meat
	1 slice bread	1 bread
	1 cup lettuce, for salad	1 vegetable
	1 tbsp. Italian dressing	1 fruit
	1 cup black coffee or tea	free
Evening	1 cup black coffee or tea	free
Snack	1 cup strawberries in	1 fruit
	½ cup skim milk	.5 milk

Day 10: 1200 Calories

Meal	Food	Exchange
Breakfast	1 cup orange juice	2 fruit
	2 slices whole-wheat toast	2 bread
	1 tsp. margarine	1 fat
	1 cup black coffee or tea	free
Mid-A.M. Snack	1 pear	1 fruit
	1 cup black coffee or tea	free
Lunch	1 cup lettuce, for salad	2 vegetable
	1 tbsp. French dressing	1 fat
	¼ cantaloupe	1 fruit
	1 cup black coffee or tea or	free
	1 bottle sugar-free beverage	free
Mid-P.M. Snack	1 cup skim milk	1 milk
	1 cup black coffee or tea	free
Dinner	4½ oz. lean ground beef patties	1.5 meat
	2 hamburger rolls	2 bread
	1 tomato	1 vegetable
	1 tsp. mayonnaise	1 fat
	½ ear of corn	1 vegetable
	1 banana	2 fruit
	1 cup black coffee or tea	free
Evening Snack	1 cup black coffee or tea	free
	1 3-inch cube angel-food cake	1 bread

Day 11: 1200 Calories

Meal	Food	Exchange
Breakfast	1 cup grapefruit juice	2 fruit
	1 bagel	2 bread
	1 tsp. margarine	1 fat
	1 cup black coffee or tea	free
Mid-A.M. Snack	½ cup pineapple	1 fruit
	1 cup black coffee or tea	free

Lunch	1 peanut butter sandwich made with 1 tsp. peanut butter	2 bread 1 fat
	1 apple	1 fruit
	1 cup black coffee or tea, or	free
	1 bottle sugar-free beverage	free
Mid-P.M. Snack	¾ cup low-fat yogurt	1 milk
	1 cup black coffee or tea	free
Dinner	4½ oz. salmon	1.5 meat
	½ cup rice	1 bread
	1 tbsp. fat-free gravy	free
	½ cup mushrooms	1 vegetable
	1 cup carrots	2 vegetable
	½ cup applesauce	1 fruit
	½ cup fruit cocktail	1 fruit
	1 cup black coffee or tea	free
Evening Snack Snack	1 cup coffee or tea	free
	⅓ cup Jell-O	1 bread
	1 cup skim milk	1 milk

Day 12: 1200 Calories

Meal	**Food**	**Exchange**
Breakfast	1 cup orange juice	2 fruit
	1 cup berries in	2 fruit
	½ cup skim milk	.5 milk
	1 cup black coffee or tea	free
Mid-A.M. Snack	½ English muffin	1 bread
	1 tsp. margarine	1 fat
	1 cup black coffee or tea	free
Lunch	10 oz. chicken-vegetable soup	2 vegetable
	3 soda crackers	1 bread
	1 apple	1 fruit
	1 cup black coffee or tea or	free
	1 bottle sugar-free beverage	free

Mid-P.M. Snack	2 graham crackers	1 bread
	1 cup black coffee or tea	free
Dinner	4½ oz. chicken in tomato sauce	1.5 meat
	made with ½ cup tomato sauce	1 vegetable
	1 cup rice	2 bread
	1 cup lettuce, for salad	1 vegetable
	1 tsp. Italian dressing	1 fat
	1 cup strawberries fresh	1 fruit
	1 cup black coffee or tea	free
Evening Snack	1 cup black coffee or tea	free
	1 hard roll	1 bread
	½ cup skim milk	.5 milk

Day 13: 1200 Calories

Meal	**Food**	**Exchange**
Breakfast	1 cup orange juice	2 fruit
	1 cup hot cereal	2 bread
	½ cup skim milk	.5 milk
	1 cup black coffee or tea	free
Mid-A.M. Snack	1 banana	1 fruit
	1 cup black coffee or tea	free
Lunch	1 cup lettuce, for salad	1 vegetable
	1 tsp. French dressing	1 fat
	2 plums	1 fruit
	1 cup black coffee or tea or	free
	1 bottle sugar-free beverage	free
Mid-P.M. Snack	1 hard roll	1 bread
	1 tsp. margarine	1 fat
	1 cup black coffee or tea	free
Dinner	4½ oz. veal	1.5 meat
	½ cup asparagus	1 vegetable
	1 cup rice	2 bread
	1 cup lettuce, for salad	1 vegetable

	1 tsp. Italian dressing	1 fat
	1 cup cranberries	1 fruit
	1 banana	2 fruit
	1 cup black coffee or tea	free
Evening Snack	1 cup black coffee or tea	free
	½ cup dry cereal	1 bread
	½ cup skim milk	.5 milk

Day 14: 1200 Calories

Meal	**Food**	**Exchange**
Breakfast	¾ cup apple juice	2 fruit
	1 English muffin	2 bread
	1 tsp. margarine	1 fat
	1 cup black coffee or tea	free
Mid-A.M. Snack	½ grapefruit	1 fruit
	1 cup black coffee or tea	free
Lunch	10 oz. onion soup	1 vegetable
	1 slice white bread	1 bread
	1 cup black coffee or tea or	free
	1 bottle sugar-free beverage	free
Mid-P.M. Snack	1 tangerine	1 fruit
	1 cup black coffee or tea	free
Dinner	4½ oz. tuna fish	1.5 meat
	1 cup macaroni	2 bread
	½ cup tomatoes	1 vegetable
	1 cup lettuce, for salad	1 vegetable
	1 tsp. French dressing	1 fat
	1 cup apple salad	1 fruit
	1 tsp. mayonnaise	1 fat
	¼ cup sherbet	1 bread
	1 cup black coffee or tea	free
Evening Snack	1 cup black coffee or tea	free
	1 cup blueberries	2 fruit
	1 cup skim milk	1 milk

Now that you have begun losing weight, let's learn how to keep that weight off while incorporating the low-fat, high-fiber eating habits into your life forever.

Beginning today, introduce the following recommendations into your normal routine. This in itself will result in a significant reduction in cholesterol, fats, sugar and sodium and an increase in dietary fiber and starch.

1. Eat smaller portions of animal products (meats, eggs, dairy products).
2. Carefully trim fat from meats before cooking.
3. Carefully trim fat from meats after cooking.
4. Eliminate butter, egg yolks, high-butterfat cheeses, whole milk, whipped cream, ice cream, sour cream, etc.
5. Substitute low-fat cheeses, egg substitutes and margarines for their counterparts.
6. Eat low-fat snacks.
7. Eliminate most frying.
8. Eat less oil, salad dressings and spreads.
9. Eliminate hardened margarines, shortening, coconut and palm oils and lard.
10. Cook meats in the oven at lower temperatures.
11. Use soy substitutes instead of meat.
12. Eliminate poultry skin and organ meat (liver, kidney, heart and brains).

There are a number of ways to increase your fiber and starch intake. Here are some tips to follow:

1. Eat more cereals.
2. Eat more bread, particularly whole wheat, bran, oatmeal.
3. Eat whole-grain bread.
4. Eat unrefined grains and cereals, especially wheat berries with seeds.
5. Eat whole fruits and vegetables, such as cauliflower, mushrooms, broccoli, onion, carrots, green pepper, corn, turnips, cabbage and radishes.
6. Eat nuts, sunflower seed kernels, fresh pineapple, etc.
7. Add unprocessed bran to salads, meat loaf, soups, etc.
8. Serve more beans, such as navy beans, pea beans, lima beans, kidney beans, pinto beans, yellow-eyed beans, black-eyed beans, split peas, chick peas, etc.

Lifetime reduction of sugar intake is a must. Here are some suggestions to follow:

1. Use less sugar in cooking.
2. Reduce sweet snacks.
3. Drink more water and less soft drinks.
4. Substitute natural fruit sugars in preparing recipes.
5. Read labels and use more sugarless products.
6. Eliminate foods high in sugar.
7. Learn to drink coffee and tea with less or no sugar.
8. Use sugarless gums and candies.

To stay on your low-fat, low-cholesterol diet for life, completely avoid the following foods.

Dairy Products
whole milk
chocolate milk
evaporated milk
condensed milk
dried whole-milk products
filled milks with coconut oil
light cream
sour cream
whipped cream
creamed cottage cheese
whole-milk yogurt
ice cream
eggnog
egg yolks
cheeses except those made from skim milk

Fats, Oils and Oil Products
margarine, heavily hydrogenated, and any hydrogenated shortening
lard
suet
bacon fat
meat drippings (before separation)
coconut oil
coconut
palm oil

mayonnaise, sauces and dressings with egg yolks, whole milk or animal
   fats
chocolate
cocoa butter
meat fats
cashew nuts
Brazil nuts

Meats
organ meats: liver, kidney and brains
beef: brisket, fillet, porterhouse steaks, T-bone steaks
pork: bacon, picnic shoulder, butt, steak, brisket, sausage
lamb and mutton: most cuts, lamb blade
poultry: duck, all skin and fat, capon, goose
fatty luncheon meats: salami, pastrami, bologna, corned beef, brisket,
   liverwurst, canned meats
frankfurters

Fish
those packed in coconut or olive oil
salted fish

Soups and Sauces
canned soups
cream soups
white sauce
béarnaise, hollandaise and other butter-based sauces
gravies
cheese sauces (except those made from skim milk)

Bakery Goods
all baked goods using butter, margarine, lard, hydrogenated shortening, cream, cream cheese, etc.
hot roll mixes
noodles
frozen breaded foods
sweet rolls
brown-and-serve rolls
dinner rolls
croissants
regular white breads

Danish pastry
éclairs, napoleons, cream puffs, etc.
sponge cakes
any baked goods made with eggs

Desserts
candy
chocolate pastries
chocolate squares
ice cream
all rich desserts
frozen cream

The key to a lifetime of healthy eating is to learn the principles of food substitution.

Avoiding the forbidden foods, many of which may have been the source of much enjoyment for you, will be a difficult undertaking. But don't be discouraged. Many products now available are low in cholesterol and saturated fats and can be substituted for their counterparts. I have also provided substitution recipes in Appendix D that I hope will be helpful. However, exercise caution, because one of the crucial aims of this program is to keep the calories from fat of all kinds to below 30 percent of the total amount of calories eaten. Direct substitution would provide a lower saturated fat and cholesterol content, but the total fat or polyunsaturated fat content would remain unaffected or might perhaps be even higher. The following foods may be substituted, provided that the total calories from fat are below 30 percent of those from all food sources and that the calories from polyunsaturates are below 10 percent. The foods in italic type are included in the recipe section of Appendix D. Experiment with some of these foods today.

Foods and Acceptable Substitutes

Dairy Products
Butter: the soft unsalted margarines, low-calorie low-fat margarines, *poly spread.*
whole milk: skim or nonfat dry milk.
whipped cream: *poly whipped cream.*
sour cream: *poly sour cream,* sour cream substitutes.

yogurt: low-fat yogurt

eggnog: Use 2 egg whites for each whole egg plus 1 whole egg for every 4 eggs requested in any eggnog recipe. Egg buds, other egg flavoring or egg substitutes may be added instead.

Eggs: Use Egg Beaters, other egg substitutes or *homemade scrambled egg substitute.*

Ice cream: *poly ice cream, orange and lemon sherbet,* ice milks, low-fat yogurt ice cream, Tofutti (soy ice cream substitute), ice banana.

Cheeses: low-fat cheddar, skim mozzarella, skim ricotta, Neufchatel, low-fat cream cheese, Saffola American, Scandic, Cheezola, Kielkase, Low Chol, Green River, Min Chol, and others. Cottage cheese: low-fat cottage cheese, pot cheese, dry-curd cottage cheese, Breeze, Lite Line and others.

Fats, Oils and Oil Products:

Margarines (Weight Watchers reduced calorie, unsalted, Diet Mazola, Mazola, Sweet-Unsalted, Fleischmann's Sweet-Unsalted, Chiffon Sweet-Unsalted), *poly spread,* Butterbud flavored oils.

Meat drippings: Separated meat drippings (tiny amount of polyunsaturated oil may be added).

Mayonnaise: *home mayonnaise.*

Chocolate: carob or a small amount of cocoa.

Peanut butter: Old-fashioned peanut butter.

Meats (see Meats on pp. 71–72 for further information):

Bacon: soy substitutes.

Ham: soy substitutes.

Corned beef brisket: Use corned beef from round or low-fat cuts.

Fish

Tuna: water packed, corn-oil packed.

Soups and Sauces

Butter sauces (béarnaise and hollandaise): Make with soft margarines.

Gravies: Use separation technique with meat drippings.

White sauces: Use soft margarines or oil with butter flavor instead of butter.

Cheese sauces: Substitute the aforementioned skim milk and low-fat cheeses.

Bakery Goods
White bread: *poly bread, poly rolls,* French bread, oatmeal bread, whole-wheat bread, English muffins, *nut bread.*
Pies: *poly pie crust.*
Cream puffs: Egg Beaters, egg substitutes.
Baked goods using eggs: Substitute Egg Beaters or other egg substitutes.

MASTERING GOOD EATING HABITS

When you go to the store today, begin reading the labels on the items you buy. Watch for the words *hydrogenated, shortening, coconut oil, palm oil, cocoa butter, hardened vegetable oil, butter, lard, cream, suet, butterfat.* If any of these words appear on the label, avoid the product. Also bypass any food labeled "cooked in vegetable fat," since the vegetable fat may be hydrogenated, or of coconut or palm oil origin. If the food item contains only slightly or partially hydrogenated oils, with most of the fat polyunsaturated, it may be used.

Beware of items that advertise as having no cholesterol or low cholesterol; before buying, check to see if they contain significant amounts of saturated or hydrogenated fats. Check the amount of cholesterol by totaling the cholesterol content in milligrams; your total intake must not exceed 250 milligrams each day. If the label does not give the cholesterol content, consult the chart in Appendix E. Since one of the key features of the 14-Day Heart-Saving Diet Plan requires that the total number of calories from fat must not exceed 30 percent of your daily caloric intake, here is a simple, rapid formula for calculating the percentage of calories from fat.

1. Read the label and look for the number of grams of fat in one serving.
2. Then look for the number of calories in one serving.
3. Multiply the number of grams of fat in one serving by 9 (the number of calories in each gram of fat) and divide by the number of calories in one serving.

For example, the label on a package of cheese may indicate that one serving contains 7 grams of fat and has 395 calories.

What percentage of the calories comes from fat?

$$\frac{\% \text{ of calories}}{\text{from fat}} = \frac{\text{grams of fat in one serving}}{\# \text{ of calories in one serving}} \times 9$$

$$\text{"} = \frac{7 \times 9 \times 100}{395}$$

$$\text{"} = \text{about } 16\%$$

This means that about 16 percent of the calories in the cheese comes from fat. If the label does not have this information, consult the charts in the Appendix.

The amount of sodium in foods is another area of great importance. Unfortunately most food labels do not indicate sodium content. It is for this reason that I have provided charts with the sodium content of most of the common foods (see Appendix E).

For the past thirty-five years Americans have been consuming vast quantities of salt in processed and frozen foods. Since the amounts vary so much in identical foods processed by different manufacturers, with few of them indicating the amounts on the labels, the Food and Drug Administration conducted consumer surveys with a view to educating manufacturers regarding the need to decrease the amount of sodium in foods, to provide low-sodium foods and to record the amount of sodium on the label. Many manufacturers have already complied and many are in the process of complying. Many new products are also appearing on the market. Congressional hearings were conducted and led to new FDA regulations, taking effect on July 1, 1985, that require all manufacturers to list the sodium content in instances in which nutritional claims are made or when a product is purported to be for a specific dietary use.

The sodium content in diets and in nutritional recommendations is conventionally given in milligrams. Sometimes it is reported in grams or millequivalents, or as salt. You can convert rapidly to milligrams by doing the following:

- If the amount of sodium is given in grams: multiply the number of grams of sodium by 1000 to convert to milligrams.
- If the amount of sodium is given in millequivalents: multiply the number of millequivalents of sodium by 23 to convert to milligrams.
- If the amount of sodium is given as milligrams of salt: multiply the number of milligrams of salt by .40 to convert to milligrams of sodium.

Defatting Technique

A very helpful tool in mastering good eating habits for life is the *defatting technique*, a method to reduce the content of fat in meats. True, the fat in meat adds flavor, but the addition of small amounts of vegetable oil will prevent much flavor loss. Just rub the oil onto the meat prior to cooking and again a few minutes before completion of the cooking process.

You are already trimming all visible fat from your meat before cooking it. But begin learning new defatting methods today. Here's how one works.

When roasting or baking meats, use an oven temperature of about 350 degrees Fahrenheit. Higher temperatures coagulate the proteins on the outside of the meat, thereby sealing in the fats, while lower temperatures assure a greater reduction of fat from the meat. Always place the meat or poultry on a rack to prevent the meat from absorbing the fat in the drippings.

Form the habit of removing all visible fat at the table. This further reduces your intake of saturated and of total fats. This habit will also be helpful when you eat out where the defatting procedure prior to cooking is not carried out.

If you take proper care in defatting, you can reduce the total fat content of meat drastically. Careful trimming alone can reduce the fat in a sirloin steak from 17 percent to 6 percent, in a veal loin chop from 10 percent to 2 percent, and in a leg of lamb from 12 percent to 4 percent.

If you inadvertently purchase a fatty canned ham, you can reduce the fat content by the following procedure: trim the fat away very carefully, then boil the ham for a while prior to baking it. After boiling, remove the ham, drain it well on absorbent towels and prepare it for baking. This will also reduce the salt content.

Separation Technique

Another helpful technique to learn in food preparation is the *separation technique*, a method for removing all the fat from meat drippings or other cooking solutions while they are still hot. It has several advantages over the usual method of placing the solution in the refrigerator until the fat hardens: (1) there is no waiting until the fat hardens; (2) more of the fat is removed; (3) separation is simpler; and (4) the amount of fat removed is readily determined. This method is also superior to spooning the oil off the top. The latter method is time consuming and results in a loss of gravy, and it is very difficult to remove all the oil.

This separation technique is done as follows: Pour the meat drippings

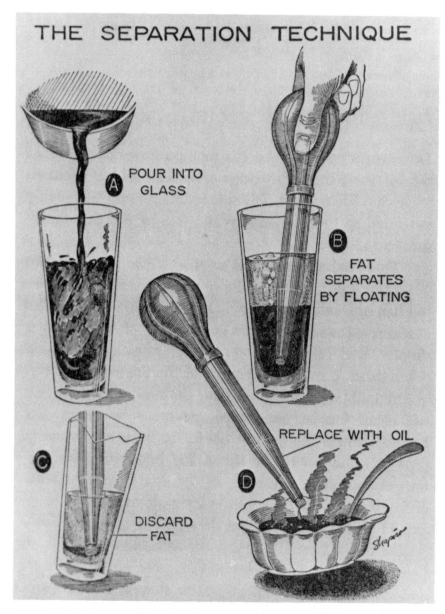

THE SEPARATION TECHNIQUE

A — POUR INTO GLASS

B — FAT SEPARATES BY FLOATING

C — DISCARD FAT

D — REPLACE WITH OIL

into a tall, clear glass so that the oil and gravy layers are easy to see. Using a bulb-type baster, depress the bulb (see drawing) and insert the tip of the injector all the way to the bottom of the glass. After the tip reaches the bottom, squeeze the bulb a little bit more in order to expel any oil trapped in the bulb during its descent through the oil layer. Slowly release the bulb and fill the baster with the gravy. The oil layer on top will merely be lowered as the gravy is removed from underneath. Lift the baster from the glass and transfer the gravy to a saucepan. Repeat this operation until about one inch of gravy remains. In order to retrieve the remaining gravy, squeeze the bulb only slightly or you will also draw in some of the oil. A little practice makes you an expert. Never attempt to remove the oil layer with the baster, as the oil will run right out of the baster.

Vegetable Oil

To avoid saturated fats in cooking and salads, always use vegetable oils. The most commonly used vegetable oils sold commercially are corn oil, cottonseed oil, safflower oil, sunflower oil, soy oil, peanut oil and sesame seed oil. An examination of the table in Appendix E shows that safflower oil contains more polyunsaturated fats and less saturated fats than the other oils, but its clinical effect in lowering blood cholesterol is similar to that of corn oil, cottonseed oil, sunflower oil and soy oil. Monounsaturates, which have a slight cholesterol-lowering effect but no cholesterol-raising effect, account for the remaining fats in these oils. The American Heart Association currently recommends that substitution of saturated fats with polyunsaturates should not exceed 10 percent of the total calories (which is in accord with the recommendations in this program), because the consequences of prolonged ingestion of large quantities are not known.

Vegetable oils keep best when refrigerated because the low temperature delays rancidity. Any air space in a container also accelerates rancidity. Therefore, if oil is purchased in large quantities, divide the oil into small containers and fill each container to the top as a further safeguard. It is also a good practice to pour the oil into smaller containers periodically, as the oil is used up.

Meats

Good lifetime eating habits also necessitate cutting down on meats. Red meats (beef, pork, lamb and veal) should only be served at one main meal each week; chicken or other lean poultry at two meals; fish at two meals and no meat at two meals. Plan your next week's menu today according to this schedule, doing your shopping in advance. Keep these recommendations in mind.

BEEF

Be very critical when buying beef. Purchase the U.S. Good and U.S. Commercial grades instead of the more expensive U.S. Prime and U.S. Choice grades, which are very high in saturated fats, usually characterized by marbling. U.S. Good beef is quite tender and comes primarily from younger animals, while U.S. Commercial beef is not very tender and comes from older animals. The percentage of fats is low in both these grades. There is an additional grade of beef on the market called U.S. Utility, but it is tough and very stringy in texture even after tenderization and maceration (pounding). The leaner, less tender steaks and roasts can be tenderized with various commercial preparations or by maceration.

Tenderizers are composed of substances called enzymes, which principally digest the fibrous tissues, making them very tender. Contrary to popular belief, these enzymes are safe to use because they are rendered harmless by cooking. The tougher cuts are frequently every bit as delicious as the choicer cuts after tenderization or maceration. Lean round steaks are delicious and only infrequently require tenderization. If you like hamburger meat, request that the butcher grind up some very lean round steak, preferably of U.S. Good grade, or select the meat yourself and instruct the butcher on how to trim it; grind it twice for greater tenderness. A tiny amount of polyunsaturated oil added to the meat will greatly enhance the flavor of the meat.

When they are well trimmed, most of the cuts have a moderate to low total fat content. Sirloin tip roast is another good choice for leanness and flavor. The saturated fat content is very high in brisket, prime rib, porterhouse steak and tenderloin (filet mignon). The defatting technique described on page 69 will greatly reduce the fat content in many of the meats.

POULTRY

Chicken is one of the leanest of meats in the young bird, but as it gets older, the fat content rises. For example, a broiler may contain only 4 percent fat while a capon may contain up to 24 percent. The fryers and roasters fall between these values. White meat has less than half the fat content of dark meat; therefore, you should buy chicken or turkey breasts more often. To roast a chicken, place it on a rack and cook at a temperature of about 325 degrees fahrenheit, as this will greatly reduce the percentage of fat. It is a good practice from a caloric point of view to avoid duck and goose. Remember, despite its succulent taste, always avoid the liver and keep it out of the stuffing or gravy, as the cholesterol content is very high. Remove the skin of poultry as it is also very high in cholesterol content.

VEAL

Veal is the leanest of the meats and should be used more frequently, but unfortunately the cost makes it almost prohibitive. The leg of veal is the leanest of the veal cuts; however, lean veal cutlets, loin and rib chops are also highly recommended. When it is properly prepared, veal ranks among the finest of gourmet dishes. Just simple trimming markedly reduces the total fat content.

PORK

Pork is an extremely nutritious food that contains all the essential amino acids and is an excellent source of iron, phosphorus, zinc and various B vitamins. Unfortunately, many people are under the misconception that pork contains far more fat than any of the other meats. This misconception probably originated over thirty years ago, when lard was in constant use and about 14 percent of the hog was used for lard. Now hogs are bred with only about 6 percent going to lard. A 3-ounce serving of cooked lean pork chops contains only about 42 milligrams of cholesterol, as compared to 58 milligrams in a 3-ounce serving of rump beef roast. Moreover, unlike beef and lamb, more than half of the fat is unsaturated.

Follow these simple rules when using pork: Buy only lean cuts; trim the visible fat carefully; and broil, bake or roast it on a rack. A ham containing about 25 percent total fat will contain less then 10 percent after careful defatting. Avoid bacon (even if it is lean to start with and cooked until crisp, the saturated fat content is very high). This does not include Canadian bacon, which is relatively low in fat content. Lean rump or shank roasts (uncooked or precooked) should be defatted as previously described. The best buy in terms of total fat content is ham legs.

LAMB AND MUTTON

Lamb and mutton are classified as lamb, yearling mutton and mutton. The cuts of lamb are further divided accorded to age: hothouse lamb (prior to weaning); spring lamb (from weaning to 5 months), and lamb. The color of lamb and mutton varies with age; lamb is reddish pink, yearling mutton is light red and mutton is a deep red.

The U.S. grading system also applies to lamb and mutton; in general, the fat content is higher in the U.S. Prime and U.S. Choice but lower in the U.S. Good and U.S. Utility grades. There is no U.S. Commercial grade for lamb and mutton.

Lean leg of lamb is the recommended cut because the fat content is quite low after defatting and roasting. Let your eye be your guide in selecting lamb, and avoid mutton except for leg of yearling mutton. If you should accidentally purchase a fatty cut of meat, use the defatting technique carefully and roast at a low temperature (325°F).

LUNCHEON MEATS

The majority of commonly purchased luncheon meats contain a very high percentage of saturated fat. Bologna, pressed meats, cooked salami, Lebanon salami, pastrami, corned beef, brisket, olive loaf, sausage meats, pickle loaf, spiced ham, pressed ham and the like are cold cuts to be avoided. Canned cold cuts and pressed cold cut products are also disallowed. Lean boiled ham, dry beef, lean Canadian bacon and lean canned ham, however, have a much lower fat content.

It is best to avoid luncheon meat completely. Use fruits and vegetables, old-fashioned peanut butter sandwiches, jelly sandwiches, the low-fat cheeses, egg salad sandwiches (made with egg substitutes) and meat substitutes. Serve one or two fish lunches each week, using salads of tuna, lobster, crabmeat or leftover baked halibut. Sardine sandwiches with lemon and onion are also good, provided you use water-packed sardines without added salt or wash the usual sardines briefly in water to remove most of the salt and then add a small amount of vegetable oil. Buy all canned fish packed in water.

Dairy Products

For healthy eating, the American Heart Association advises that you cut down on dairy products. Dairy products are notorious for their high content of saturated fat. These products, which include milk, cream, butter, cheese, ice cream, sour cream, whipped cream and so on, make a significant contribution to the total saturated fat content of the American diet. (See Appendix E for an overall picture of the saturated and polyunsaturated fat content of the various dairy products.)

It is important that you restrict your intake of all dairy products with the exception of skim milk, nonfat milk, low-fat cheeses and homemade yogurt. Milk is an important food nutritionally; it is an important source of minerals, protein and some vitamins that are necessary for good nutrition. Nonfat dry milk and skim milk contain all the nutrients of whole milk minus the high content of saturated fat.

Don't expect an inveterate milk drinker to switch to skim or nonfat milk overnight. The change must be very gradual, over many months. One recommendation is to mix one quart of whole milk to one quart of 2 percent milk, resulting in 3 percent milk. Drink this for about two months, then switch to 2 percent milk for a few months. Try switching further to 1 percent milk and see how it goes. If you have difficulty, go back to 2 percent. Vitamin A is not restored in commercial skim or nonfat dry milk; therefore, an adequate intake of foods high in vitamin A or taking vitamin supplements is necessary. One undesirable characteristic of skim milk is its lack of body, but this can be improved by adding some nonfat dry milk. Serve these low-fat milks with added maple, vanilla, maple-vanilla or cocoa. Whenever a recipe calls for whole milk, use nonfat or skim milk instead. In most instances you will find that you cannot tell the difference in the final product.

Avoid cream and ice cream products, because they contain a very high percentage of saturated fats. Although ice milk has a lower saturated fat content than ice cream, you should avoid it because the amount of fat is still too high. A delightful substitute for whipped cream can be made easily from nonfat dry milk and a tiny amount of unflavored vegetable oil (see Appendix D). This is excellent for strawberry shortcake, pudding, cakes, gelatins and so on. A good substitute ice cream (poly ice cream) that I developed can easily be prepared in many flavors using nonfat dry milk and a small amount of unflavored oil. The only equipment required is an electric mixer (see Appendix D). The poly ice cream has the following properties: the oil does not separate out, there are no ice crystals formed and it keeps for a long time when frozen. It must not be made with corn oil, which leaves an undesirable corn aftertaste. A tasty new soy milk ice cream substitute called Tofutti is also currently available. Beware of some vegetable oil "ice cream substitutes" that are made with hydrogenated oils. Use more of the homemade sherbets that are delicious, easy to prepare and do not have any fat calories that you have to worry about (see Appendix D).

Butter is one of the most important foods to avoid because it contains over 80 percent fat, mostly saturated. Margarines in general consist of 80 percent fat, about 16 percent water, 2 to 3 percent nonfat milk solids and preservatives. The fat, however, is made of vegetable oils, primarily corn, soybean or cottonseed oil, but safflower, peanut and sunflower oils are also used. There are two types of margarine to avoid: those made with neutral lard and those with a high degree of hydrogenation to make them hard. Margarine should be low in hydrogenated (hardened) fats; high in polyunsaturates; low in saturates; have a mild, butterlike taste with a pleasant flavor; be low in sodium; and have a smooth spreadability. Margarines like Mazzola unsalted, Fleischman's Unsalted and Chiffon sweet unsalted appear to satisfy these criteria. Since margarines are high in total fats, use them sparingly. The poly butter spread is very tasty and can be substituted for butter or margarine. This spread can be made simply with an electric mixer. It is very low in saturated fat and is more economical than butter or margarine. It can be used on toast, as a dip for crab and lobster in place of butter sauce, in mashed potatoes and vegetables, with egg substitutes, or as a garlic butter, Roquefort butter, horseradish butter, anchovy butter and so on (see Appendix D). Unfortunately it cannot be used for frying because the milk solids make it stick to the pan.

Until recently, of the hundreds of kinds of cheeses made in this country and imported from all over the world, very few were low in saturated fats and cholesterol. Many low-fat, low-cholesterol cheeses are currently available, including low-fat cottage cheese, pot cheese, dry curd cottage cheese, Breeze, Lite line, low-fat cheddar, skim mozzarella, skim ricotta, Neufchatel low-fat cream cheese, Saffola American, Scandic, Cheezola, Kiel-kase, Low Chol, Green River, Min Chol and others. Avoid creamed cottage cheese, which contains about 5 percent fat, as compared to "nonfat" cottage cheese containing less than 1 percent fat. Cottage cheese is very useful as a base in making dips and dressings for potatoes by mixing it in a blender with a little skim milk. It has also been successfully used as a substitute in making cheesecake and is used in making homemade scrambled egg substitutes. When eating spaghetti, go easy on the grated Romano or Parmesan cheese. Some of the commercial yogurts are unsatisfactory, as they are made from whole milk and fat solids. Concentrate on the skim milk yogurts or make the yogurt yourself at home, using skim milk. A delightful substitute for sour cream that tastes very much like the real thing is excellent for dips, salads, baked potato dressing and in many recipes. It uses yogurt that was strained through cheesecloth with gelatin added (see Appendix D). A yogurt spread can be made by straining yogurt through cheesecloth. This is excellent on toast, as a shrimp dip and as a dressing.

What About Eggs?

There has been much confusion about the use of eggs in the diet. The truth of the matter is that only egg whites can be used, because the yolk of one egg contains about 240 milligrams of cholesterol, which approximates the total daily amount of cholesterol that is permissible (250 milligrams).

You can eat one egg if you totally eliminate all other sources of cholesterol on that day.

Whenever a recipe calls for a whole egg, try substituting two egg whites instead. If the recipe calls for several eggs, use one or two whole eggs and two egg whites for each additional egg requested. Use Egg Beaters or other egg substitutes in your recipes, with or without egg whites. French toast and spong cakes prepared with Egg Beaters taste identical to those prepared with whole eggs. A satisfactory taste for scrambled eggs, cream puffs and soufflés can also be achieved with egg substitutes.

Substitute scrambled eggs can be made with egg whites mixed with cottage cheese or nonfat dried milk and a dash of yellow food coloring added. Egg flavorings like Egg Buds may be added for additional flavor.

Fish

Most Americans eat too much meat and not enough fish. To keep slim and healthy for the rest of your life, remember to increase your consumption of seafood. Seafood is the ideal substitute for meat because its fat content is low, the polyunsaturated fat content is high, the saturated fat content is low and the protein content is high. Three new studies published in the May 1985 issue of *New England Journal of Medicine* add support to the beneficial effects of fish consumption in preventing cardiovascular and other diseases. In one study conducted in the Netherlands for twenty years on 852 middle-aged men, it was found that fatal heart attacks were 50 percent lower among those who ate at least one ounce of fish per day than those who ate no fish at all. They also concluded that eating only two fish meals each week may be of value in preventing coronary artery disease. Fish also provides an abundance of vitamins, minerals and necessary chemical elements, including iodine, iron, phosphorus, calcium and magnesium.

Fish is divided into two main groups: the lean fish and the fat fish. The former are characterized by white flesh, contain a small percentage of fat and are low in calories. The latter fish have flesh that varies in shade from red to white and are relatively higher in fat content and calories. Since all fish fats are low in saturated fats and high in polyunsaturated fats, the primary problem in eating fat fishes is the calorie count. There are relatively few fat fishes used as food, the common ones being salmon, tuna, pompano, mackerel, sardines, eels, smelt, herring, trout and white fish. Fish, particularly the fatty ones, contain a special class of polyunsaturated fatty acids called omega-3 fatty acids, which significantly lowers blood cholesterol and triglycerides.

Many people, unfortunately, do not eat seafood because they do not know how to handle or cook it. Others are under the misconception that fish is hard to digest. Fish flesh is actually easier to digest than animal flesh, because the proteins in fish are of the globular, easy-to-digest type. Fish is only cooked to bring out its flavor and to kill bacteria and parasites, not to render it more tender, since it is already tender in the raw state. If fish is overcooked, it becomes leathery and difficult to chew.

Fish is sold in various forms (cuts): *Whole* fish are sold as caught. *Drawn* fish have only the insides removed. Both have to be scaled, and head, tail and fins removed. *Dressed* or *pan-ready* fish have the insides, head, tail and scales removed. *Fillets* are the sides of dressed fish cut lengthwise from the backbone and are boneless and ready to cook. If the fillets from both sides are joined at the belly, they take on a butterfly shape and are called *butterfly fillets. Fish sticks* are fillets cut into small portions usually an inch wide and three inches long. *Fish steaks* are cross slices obtained from the larger fishes, such as halibut, swordfish and salmon.

Purchase fresh fish because it spoils more rapidly than meat. Look for the following characteristics when purchasing fish: eyes that are clear and bulging; gills that have a reddish-pink look; scales that glisten and are strongly adherent; flesh that is resilient (springs back when gently pressed, and finger impressions readily disappear); and fish that is free of slime and strong odors.

The quicker you cook fish after purchase, the tastier it is. Pack it in ice, store it in the coldest part of the refrigerator and use it as soon as possible. Prior to freezing fish, place the fish in a plastic bag and fill the bag with cold tap water for freshwater fish and slightly salted water for saltwater fish so that it is totally immersed. Fish stored in this manner tastes as fresh as the day it was frozen.

SHELLFISH

You can eat shellfish. Shellfish have always been condemned in low-cholesterol diets because they contain a significant amount of cholesterol, but recent findings indicate that the presence in shellfish of a class of polyunsaturated fatty acids called omega-3 fatty acids appears to offset the effect of the cholesterol. This means that shellfish can be used moderately, but your consumption of it should not exceed four ounces in a day. The total fat content in shellfish, however, is quite low, and it provides many of the minerals that are important to health and growth.

There are over three hundred different species of shrimp around the world, with shells varying in color from green to brown to pink to white to reddish brown. But one thing is common to all: they turn pinkish red during cooking.

Shrimp are sold according to size; the following chart categorizes them according to size and the number of each to a pound before and after shelling.

Size	Raw, Unshelled	Raw, Shelled
small	50–60	65–75
medium	40–50	50–60
large	30–38	38–48
jumbo	18–25	25–33
colossal	8–12	15–20

There is a 25 percent loss in weight after shelling and an additional loss of 25 percent following cooking. Thawed shrimp should be cooked within one day of purchase and after being cooked should not be refrigerated more than three to four days. Freezing cooked shrimp should be accomplished by placing them in a plastic bag or plastic container and immersing them in the solution they were cooked in. This maintains them in a fresh, succulent state.

Deveining is a matter of personal preference; some do and some don't. This "vein" located along the outer curve of the shrimp is often referred to as the sand vein because the dark substance within it has a somewhat gritty or sandy texture. The sand vein is not a vein at all but the intestinal tract of the shrimp. The gritty material is partially digested plankton that has been eaten by the shrimp.

Lobsters are available live, cooked in the shell, as fresh or frozen lobster meat and in cans. A live lobster weighs three-quarters of a pound to three or more pounds, with the meat coming from the tail and claws. Live northern or Maine lobsters can be purchased for shipment to all parts of the country. Do not confuse Maine lobsters with rock lobsters, which only have marketable tails and are imported from South Africa, Australia and New Zealand. These tails run from four ounces to a pound each.

Crabs include the hardshell or blue crab from the Atlantic, the Dungeness crab from the Pacific and the King and Queen crab from Pacific Alaskan waters. Another popular dish is softshell crabs. These are really blue crabs after they have shed their shells (molting stage). Crabs are available live, cooked in the shell, as fresh or frozen meat and in cans. Pasteurized crabmeat is also available. The meat is available from the claws (claw meat), the larger muscles (lump meat) and the remaining meat (flake meat). The King crabs are gigantic and may weigh from three to twenty pounds.

Dining Out

Eating out need not present a problem in adhering to your diet plan. When you are invited out, be unobtrusive, tactful and uncomplaining to avoid offending your host or hostess. Nonetheless, be sure to:

1. Trim away all visible fat and select lean portions.
2. Concentrate more on items that are low in fat.
3. Eat moderately. For example, select salads, fruits, gelatin and vegetables, and only a small portion of the meat.
4. Avoid sauces and rich desserts.
5. If it is a formal affair, eat smaller portions and select the least fatty meat, such as chicken instead of prime ribs. It is socially acceptable to refuse the dessert.
6. Pass up the hors d'oeuvres or select the nonfatty ones.

At restaurants, make selections that adhere as closely as possible to the principles you learned in the 14-Day Heart-Saving Menu Plan. Of course, your decisions will differ according to the menus offered at different restaurants.

1. If you eat out on a regular basis, select a restaurant that fits your needs and eat there often.
2. Choose whole wheat, French or oatmeal bread and hard rolls over hot rolls and biscuits.
3. Don't use butter. Ask for soft margarine, but if it is unavailable, use jelly or honey on your bread.
4. Try Chinese, Japanese, Mexican, Lebanese, Greek and Italian restaurants. Foods from these cultures are low in fat and cholesterol and provide ample vegetable, grain and starch foods, with less emphasis on meats and other high-cholesterol, high-fat foods. Avoid those dishes that emphasize meat or dairy products. If you don't know, ask the waiter what a particular item on the menu consists of.

RECOMMENDED STAPLES

Go out and buy some of these recommended staples, many of which will be used frequently in this program:

    ground bran
    beans and dried peas of all types
    bulghur wheat
    barley

nuts (pecans, walnuts, hazelnuts, filberts, pistachios, almonds, etc.)
raisins
sunflower seeds
rice (white, brown, wild)
bread (whole wheat, French, homemade, English muffins, oatmeal, pita, etc.)
graham crackers and oatmeal cookies
bean sprouts
dried mushrooms
tomato sauce, paste and tomatoes
peanut butter, sesame seed butter
cornmeal
egg substitute and food coloring
bouillon cubes (chicken and beef)
spices (see chapter 5)
pasta (spaghetti, macaroni, etc.)
cereals (oatmeal, shredded wheat, bran, mixed grain, etc.)

The principles and techniques presented in this chapter constitute your eating prescription for a healthy heart. Follow this program as if your life depended on it, because it very well may.

Chapter Four

The 14-Day Heart-Saving

Quit-Smoking Plan

> *Habit is habit, and not to be flung out of the window by any man, but coaxed downstairs a step at a time.*
>
> —Mark Twain

The 14-Day Heart-Saving Stop-Smoking Plan is designed to help you stop smoking in fourteen days. If you are successful, you will have eliminated one of the major contributing causes of heart attack.

Yet there is really no easy way to stop smoking. The key to success is motivation, because without it the chances of stopping are very slim. But how can one become properly motivated? The answer is through education. As Alexander Pope wrote, " 'Tis education forms the common mind: / Just as the twig is bent, the tree's inclined." Certainly the best-motivated people are those who have been stricken with a serious illness and know that if they don't stop smoking they may die or become invalids. They have become motivated by seeing the facts and experiencing fear, an extreme form of education. Still, the likelihood of acquiring a serious illness or dying because of smoking is very high. So don't wait until you must stop smoking. Become aware of the hazards of smoking and the benefits of quitting now.

SMOKER'S SELF-AWARENESS PROFILE

Smoking has been described as an unconscious act, because smokers very often light a cigarette without thinking about it or without even realizing they are doing it. The following Smoker's Self-Awareness Profile is comprised of two tests to help you become more conscious of the reasons you smoke, how you feel about smoking and why you want to quit. Answer each questionnaire on a separate sheet of paper and determine your score on each one. Armed with this self-knowledge, you will be better prepared to exchange your smoking habit for a nonsmoking habit.

Test 1: Why Do You Smoke?

Here are some statements made by people to describe what they get out of smoking cigarettes. How often do you feel this way when smoking them? Circle one number for each statement.

Important: Answer every question.

	ALWAYS	FRE-QUENTLY	OCCA-SIONALLY	SELDOM	NEVER
A. I smoke cigarettes in order to keep myself from slowing down.	5	4	3	2	1
B. Handling a cigarette is part of the enjoyment of smoking it.	5	4	3	2	1
C. Smoking cigarettes is pleasant and relaxing.	5	4	3	2	1
D. I light up a cigarette when I feel angry about something.	5	4	3	2	1
E. When I have run out of cigarettes I find it almost unbearable until I can get them.	5	4	3	2	1
F. I smoke cigarettes automatically without even being aware of it.	5	4	3	2	1
G. I smoke cigarettes to stimulate me, to perk myself up.	5	4	3	2	1
H. Part of the enjoyment of smoking a cigarette comes from the steps I take to light up.	5	4	3	2	1
I. I find cigarettes pleasurable.	5	4	3	2	1
J. When I feel uncomfortable or upset about something, I light up a cigarette.	5	4	3	2	1
K. I am very much aware of the fact when I am not smoking a cigarette.	5	4	3	2	1
L. I light up a cigarette without realizing I still have one burning in the ashtray.	5	4	3	2	1
M. I smoke cigarettes to give me a "lift."	5	4	3	2	1
N. When I smoke a cigarette, part of the enjoyment is watching the smoke as I exhale it.	5	4	3	2	1
O. I want a cigarette most when I am comfortable and relaxed.	5	4	3	2	1
P. When I feel "blue" or want to take my mind off cares and worries, I smoke cigarettes.	5	4	3	2	1
Q. I get a real gnawing hunger for a cigarette when I haven't smoked for a while.	5	4	3	2	1
R. I've found a cigarette in my mouth and didn't remember putting it there.	5	4	3	2	1

How to score:
1. Enter the numbers you have circled to the test questions in the spaces below, putting the number you have circled to Question A over line A, to Question B over line B, etc.
2. Total the 3 scores on each line to get your totals. For example, the sum of your scores over lines A, G, and M gives you your score on Stimulation—lines B, H, and N give the score on Handling, etc.

Totals

_____ A	+ _____ G	+ _____ M	= _____ Stimulation
_____ B	+ _____ H	+ _____ N	= _____ Handling
_____ C	+ _____ I	+ _____ O	= _____ Pleasurable Relaxation
_____ D	+ _____ J	+ _____ P	= _____ Crutch: Tension Reduction
_____ E	+ _____ K	+ _____ Q	= _____ Craving: Psychological Addiction
_____ F	+ _____ L	+ _____ R	= _____ Habit

Scores can vary from 3 to 15. Any score 11 and above is high; any score 7 and below is low. Learn from Part 2 what your scores mean.

What Your Scores on Test 1 Tell About Why You Smoke
What kind of smoker are you? What do you get out of smoking? What does it do for you? This test is designed to provide you with a score on each of 6 factors which describe many people's smoking. Your smoking may be well characterized by only one of these factors, or by a combination of factors.

A score of 11 or above on any factor indicates that this factor is an important source of satisfaction for you. The higher your score (15 is the highest), the more important a particular factor is in your smoking and the more useful the discussion of that factor can be in your attempt to quit.

1. Stimulation
If you score high or fairly high on this factor, it means that you are one of those smokers who are stimulated by the cigarette—you feel that it helps wake you up, organizes your energies, and keeps you going. If you try to give up smoking, you may want a safe substitute (a brisk walk or moderate exercise, for example), whenever you feel the urge to smoke.

2. Handling
Handling things can be satisfying, but there are many ways to keep your hands busy without lighting up or playing with a cigarette. Why not toy with a pen or pencil? Or try doodling. Or play with a coin, a piece of jewelry, or some other harmless object.

3. Accentuation of pleasure—pleasurable relaxation
It is not always easy to find out whether you use the cigarette to feel good, that is, get real, honest pleasure out of smoking (Factor 3) or keep from feeling so bad (Factor 4). About two-thirds of smokers score high or fairly high on accentuation

of pleasure, and about half of those also score as high or higher on reduction of negative feelings.

Those who do get real pleasure out of smoking often find that an honest consideration of the harmful effects of their habit is enough to help them quit.

4. Reduction of negative feelings, or "crutch"

Many smokers use the cigarette as a kind of crutch in moments of stress or discomfort, and on occasion it may work; the cigarette is sometimes used as a tranquilizer. But the heavy smoker, the person who tries to handle severe personal problems by smoking many times a day, is apt to discover that cigarettes do not help him deal with his problems effectively.

5. "Craving" or psychological addiction

Quitting smoking is difficult for the person who scores high on this factor—that of psychological addiction. For him, the craving for the next cigarette begins to build up the moment he puts one out.

Giving up cigarettes may be so difficult and cause so much discomfort that once he does quit, he will find it easy to resist the temptation to go back to smoking because he knows that some day he will have to go through the same agony again.

6. Habit

This kind of smoker is no longer getting much satisfaction from his cigarettes. He just lights them frequently without even realizing he is doing so. He may find it easy to quit and stay off if he can break the habit patterns he has built up. Cutting down gradually may be quite effective if there is a change in the way the cigarettes are smoked and the conditions under which they are smoked. The key to success is becoming aware of each cigarette you smoke. This can be done by asking yourself, "Do I really want this cigarette?" You may be surprised at how many you do not want.

Test 2: Do You Want to Change Your Smoking Habits?

For each statement, circle the number that most accurately indicates how you feel. For example, if you completely agree with the statement, circle 4, if you agree somewhat, circle 3, etc.
Important: Answer every question.

	COMPLETELY AGREE	SOMEWHAT AGREE	SOMEWHAT DISAGREE	COMPLETELY DISAGREE
A. Cigarette smoking might give me a serious illness.	4	3	2	1
B. My cigarette smoking sets a bad example for others.	4	3	2	1
C. I find cigarette smoking to be a messy kind of habit.	4	3	2	1
D. Controlling my cigarette smoking is a challenge to me.	4	3	2	1
E. Smoking causes shortness of breath.	4	3	2	1
F. If I quit smoking cigarettes it might influence others to stop.	4	3	2	1
G. Cigarettes cause damage to clothing and other personal property.	4	3	2	1
H. Quitting smoking would show that I have willpower.	4	3	2	1
I. My cigarette smoking will have a harmful effect on my health.	4	3	2	1
J. My cigarette smoking influences others close to me to take up or continue smoking.	4	3	2	1
K. If I quit smoking, my sense of taste or smell would improve.	4	3	2	1
L. I do not like the idea of feeling dependent on smoking.	4	3	2	1

How to score:
1. Enter the numbers you have circled to the test questions in the spaces below, putting the number you have circled to Question A over line A, to Question B over line B, etc.
2. Total the 3 scores across on each line to get your totals. For example, the sum of your scores over lines A, E, and I gives you your score on Health—lines B, F, and J give the score on Example, etc.

Totals

$$\underline{\hspace{2cm}}_{\text{A}} + \underline{\hspace{2cm}}_{\text{E}} + \underline{\hspace{2cm}}_{\text{I}} = \underline{\hspace{2cm}}_{\text{Health}}$$

$$\underline{\hspace{2cm}}_{\text{B}} + \underline{\hspace{2cm}}_{\text{F}} + \underline{\hspace{2cm}}_{\text{J}} = \underline{\hspace{2cm}}_{\text{Example}}$$

$$\underline{\hspace{2cm}}_{\text{C}} + \underline{\hspace{2cm}}_{\text{G}} + \underline{\hspace{2cm}}_{\text{K}} = \underline{\hspace{2cm}}_{\text{Esthetics}}$$

$$\underline{\hspace{2cm}}_{\text{D}} + \underline{\hspace{2cm}}_{\text{H}} + \underline{\hspace{2cm}}_{\text{L}} = \underline{\hspace{2cm}}_{\text{Mastery}}$$

Scores can vary from 3 to 12. Any score 9 and above is high; any score 6 and below is low. Learn from Part 2 what your scores mean.

What Your Scores on Test 2 Tell About Your Smoking Habits
Why do you want to quit smoking? Are your reasons strong enough for you to make the effort to quit? Do you have enough reasons? This is something only you can decide.

Four common reasons for wanting to quit smoking cigarettes are: Concern over the effects on health; desire to set an example for others; recognition of the unpleasant aspects of smoking; and desire to exercise self-control.

A score of 9 or above in one of these categories indicates that this is one of the most important reasons why you may want to quit.

1. Health
Research during the past 10 or 15 years has shown that cigarette smoking can be harmful to health. Knowing this, many people have recently stopped smoking and many others are considering it. If your score on the health factor is 9 or above, the health hazards of smoking may be enough to make you want to quit now.

2. Example
Some people stop smoking because they want to set a good example for others. Parents do it to make it easier for their children to resist starting to smoke; doctors do it to influence their patients; teachers want to help their students; sports stars want to set an example for their young fans; husbands want to influence their wives, and vice versa.

Such examples are an important influence on our behavior. Research shows that almost twice as many high school students smoke if both parents are smokers compared to those whose parents are nonsmokers or former smokers.

If your score is low (6 or less), perhaps you do not appreciate how important your example could be.

3. Esthetics
People who score high, that is, 9 or above, in this category, recognize and are disturbed by some of the unpleasant aspects of smoking. The smell of stale smoke

on their clothing, bad breath, and stains on their fingers and teeth might be reason enough to consider breaking the habit.

4. Mastery (self-control)

If you score 9 or above on this factor, you are bothered by the knowledge that you cannot control your desire to smoke. You are not your own master. Awareness of this challenge to your self-control may make you want to quit.

REASONS FOR LIKING AND DISLIKING CIGARETTES

Take two blank sheets of paper and title one "Why I Like Smoking" and the other sheet "Why I Dislike Smoking." Describe in your own words why you like or dislike smoking. Since knowledge is power, self-knowledge will give you power over yourself, the ability to master and overcome the smoking habit.

THE I QUIT CALENDAR

Now take a look at the I Quit Calendar on page 89. There are no dates on it, but it is designed to represent two full weeks. This program is planned to be completed in fourteen days. The fourteenth day is the I Quit Day. You can pick the day of the week you want to start (the first of the week, perhaps a Monday when you might be more relaxed), or perhaps you'd rather start by selecting a "quit day" and working backward toward day 1. Buy a package of gold stars with adhesive and award yourself a star in the space provided on the calendar, or merely color in the star with a yellow crayon.

Read each day's instructions at the first opportunity—before breakfast if possible—and follow them faithfully. Quitting smoking is a conscious act that requires conscious self-discipline, so make it a rule to stick to the program as closely as possible. Set a plan for each day even if you should decide to repeat the same plan for more than one day.

You may suffer a relapse, no matter how good your intentions. *Don't regard any setback as a sign of failure.* It isn't easy to quit smoking, but you can do it! If the first quit period isn't successful, go back to the last day of the plan you were successful with and pick it up from there.

I Quit Calendar

S	M	T	W	T	F	S

DAY 1

Start being conscious of not smoking.

1. *Change your brand of cigarettes, and buy only one pack at a time.* Today throw out all your cigarettes even if you have ten cartons of them. Now buy one pack of another brand—one that you don't particularly like. Don't buy another pack until you've smoked the first. Since smoking is an unconscious act, to quit you must become conscious of the act of smoking. Then apply your consciousness to developing the habit of not smoking. The first step is to be aware of every pack you smoke by making it an act of conscious will to buy a pack of cigarettes. Here's how.

2. *Rate your need for each cigarette on a smoking record.* If you're like most smokers, you probably smoke a lot more often than you really feel like smoking. To prove this to yourself, take a sheet of ruled paper and write the following headings across the top of the sheet: "Cigarette," "Time of Day," "Activity," "Feeling," "Need Rating from 1 to 3."

   Now rate your need for a cigarette as follows: A 1 would mean you feel you need the cigarette very much and couldn't function without it. A 2 could mean you want the cigarette, but not that badly. A 3 would mean that you really could do without it. Below "Cigarette," write whether it is your first of the day, second, third and so on. The first few lines might look as follows:

Cigarette	Time of Day	Activity	Feeling	Need Rating from 1 to 3
1	8:45	waiting for bus	bored	3
2	9:20	on telephone with customer	irritated	1
3	10:30	coffee break	relaxed	2

Fill out the Smoking Record before you light up each cigarette. Remember that the purpose of this exercise is to make you conscious of the decision to smoke.

Keep this Smoking Record stuffed inside the cigarette package or wrapped around it with a rubber band, so that it will always be handy and you can't reach for a cigarette without seeing it and filling it out.

I'm not asking you to start cutting down today, but you may be surprised to see how often, after you've consciously analyzed your desire to smoke a cigarette, you'll decide not to smoke it after all.

Here are some ways to become conscious of not smoking:

Put up an I Want to Quit poster. Make a poster with large letters saying **I Want to Quit**. Put this up where you will see it often—on the refrigerator or on the wall of your office.

Don't clean out your ashtrays. This is another consciousness-raising exercise. As the butts pile up, you'll become acutely aware of just how many cigarettes you've smoked during the day.

Slow down your smoking ritual. Before you quit smoking, try wrapping your cigarette pack with a sheet of paper like a Christmas present. Every time you want a cigarette, unwrap the pack and write down what you are doing, how you feel and how important this cigarette is to you. After you get a craving for a cigarette, never smoke until three minutes have passed since you got the urge. Instead, take a drink or phone a friend until the craving subsides. Finally, smoke only half of each cigarette.

Make a list. List the following benefits on an index card and read it when you feel like smoking.

1. Decreased risk of heart attack.
2. Increased production of good cholesterol.
3. Decreased risk of lung disease.
4. Less coughing.
5. Less carbon monoxide in the blood.
6. Food tastes better.

7. Teeth are whiter.
8. More money to spend.
9. More wind for exercise.
10. Fresher breath.

Change your pattern until you quit. Make yourself a "smoking corner" that is far from anything interesting. If you like to smoke with others, always smoke alone. If you like to smoke alone, always smoke with others, preferably if they are nonsmokers. Never smoke while watching television.

Make quitting a game. Bet with someone that you can quit. Put the cigarette money in a jar each morning and forfeit it if you smoke. You keep the money if you don't smoke by the end of the week. Try to extend this period so that you get a bigger and bigger jackpot.

Talk to your doctor. If you are depressed or have physical symptoms that might be related to your smoking, relieve your mind by discussing this with your physician. It is easier to quit when you know your health status.

DAY 2

Start cutting down on your smoking.
Keep up your Smoking Record, but today when you rate a cigarette a 3, don't smoke it. Try a stick of gum or celery or a carrot stick. Or get up for a stretch or a stroll.

Stack up on low-calorie snacks.
Smoking satisfies what psychologists call an oral need. As another way of satisfying this oral need, stock up on celery, carrot sticks or sugarless gum, and keep them handy. Don't start eating cookies, candy or peanuts, or you will soon have a weight problem as difficult to overcome as your smoking habit. If coffee and cigarettes go together for you, try switching to tea, a soft drink or juice when you would normally drink coffee.

Take a walk.
Another way to relax is by taking a twenty-minute walk after dinner, or begin an aerobic exercise program from chapter 2 instead of smoking your afterdinner cigarette. It'll help you digest your food and give you a chance to fill your lungs with clean fresh air instead of smoke. Make moderate exercise part of your quitting regimen. You may grow to like the feeling of peace and relaxation it brings and decide to keep it up after you've quit smoking.

Doctors have noted that many patients who smoke seem to have "given up on their bodies," especially those whose work is basically sedentary. Remember what pleasure you used to take in your physical prowess? Even if you were not particularly athletic, you enjoyed physical activity. You can regain that kind of pleasure, that kind of physical confidence, but you'll need clean lungs to feel that way again.

DAY 3

Cut down more on your smoking.
Are you still keeping your Smoking Record? Don't get out of the habit of doing so. Remember, as you smoke fewer cigarettes, you'll have a better check on which cigarettes are the hardest for you to give up. Have you been successful in eliminating any of your number-3-rated cigarettes? If so, try today to skip some of your number-2-rated cigarettes.

Begin breathing exercises.
Professionally designed and tested deep-breathing exercises, practiced morning and evening, will help relieve tensions and combat the urge to smoke. Here are two that can be done in your office, at school or at home.

Supine Breathing Exercise

1. Lie on the floor in a relaxed position, with your knees bent and your feet flat on the floor.

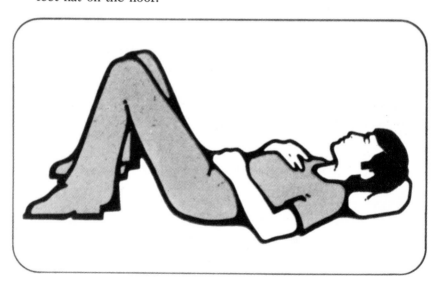

2. Keep your lower back flat, not arched. To be certain that your back is not arched, press it against the floor a couple of times.
3. Breathe normally. Place your hands just below your rib cage so you can feel your diaphragm lift and drop.
4. Now when you are ready to begin, inhale normally, then exhale with a whispered *ahhhhhh*. When most of your breath is gone, finish exhaling by counting out slowly *1-2-3-4*-etc. until you have exhaled every last ounce of air and are beginning to feel a slight strain.
5. As you inhale again, your diaphragm should spring up. Keep trying to increase your count before inhaling.
6. Do this exercise ten times in the morning and ten times at night as a relaxation or distraction ritual.

Here's another simple breathing exercise that can be done standing up:

Standing Breathing Exercise
Stand with your feet apart and comfortable. Now close your eyes and let your head bend forward. Drop your head further now, and slowly inhale through your nose. Draw your breath deeply into your abdomen, allowing your abdomen to expand and your head to rise slowly as you inhale. Hold your breath gently, then exhale slowly. Breathe out through your nose. Take your time and repeat this breathing exercise at whatever pace feels comfortable. Do it slowly. Stop for a few moments if you get dizzy. Take your time, and when you feel ready to stop, just slowly open your eyes.

Try another, simpler breathing exercise as a substitute for a cigarette. A lot of people find that the action of breathing in and out deeply three or four times makes them feel better and more relaxed (with a fresher taste in their mouths than if they'd smoked a cigarette).

Pace yourself on a time basis.
Pick a particular time of the day when you generally smoke and try to go for a definite, scheduled period without smoking—say one hour if you're a heavy smoker, two hours if you're a moderate smoker or a half-day if you're a light smoker.

Don't forget to take a walk and do your aerobic exercise.
Don't forget, you can exercise self-control over smoking. You don't smoke on a bus or in the theater, do you? Why? Because you accept the externally imposed restraint and you live with it. If you can accept an externally imposed restraint, you can accept an internally imposed restraint as well. In other words, you can tell yourself to stop smoking. Also, the urge to smoke will eventually go away whether you smoke or not. The craving for

nicotine, the urge to light up, will pass if you don't smoke. It will reassert itself again later on, but less forcefully, and if you don't give in, the next urge will be easier to resist.

DAY 4

Take a good look at the I Quit poster.

Imagine yourself as someone who successfully quit smoking. You'll be in good company. A lot of famous people have quit smoking, and a lot of ordinary people have too.

Quitting was hard for many, but for some it went smoothly. They were all prey to pressures, tensions and temptations, but they overcame them to join the growing majority of ex-smokers who have made a commitment to quit.

Pick a situation in which to quit smoking.

Probably the best situation to pick would be one in which you would not be too tempted to smoke anyway, say walking somewhere or working in the kitchen.

But maybe you'd rather pick a tougher situation, say at a meeting or at a party.

Pretend there's a No Smoking sign in the room or nailed to a tree, and don't smoke for the duration of the particular activity you've chosen. Or try not smoking during the odd- or even-numbered hours of the clock.

Once you've learned you can control your smoking urge in one situation, try others. You'll find that in many of those situations in which you feel you just "have to have a cigarette," you really don't need one at all.

Continue to keep your Smoking Record.

By now many of your cigarettes should be rated 2 instead of 1, since you should be gaining considerable mastery over your smoking urge. Don't kid yourself and start rating cigarettes 1 that should be rated 2 or 3.

Remember, you could live without that cigarette if you had to, say if your arms were full of packages or you were skiing or swimming. Tell yourself you can't smoke those cigarettes. Try to quit smoking all of those 2-rated cigarettes today.

Do your breathing exercises. Take your walk. Think about quitting cold tomorrow.

Are you making good progress? Have you really cut your cigarette consumption? Are your feeling good? Feeling confident? If so, maybe you're ready to quit cold turkey. Cold turkey means stopping abruptly. You do not smoke any more cigarettes—not even one. If so, skip to day 7, and move the 7 on your I Quit Calendar to tomorrow.

If you feel hesitant, stay with the program and go on to Day 5 tomorrow.

DAY 5

Put away your matches and lighters.
If you have to ask someone for a light every time you want to smoke, you'll gain precious minutes in which to change your mind.

Keep up your Smoking Record. Today you should be smoking no number-2-rated cigarettes, and your number-1-rated cigarettes should have diminished to just a few.

Better yet, throw away your cigarettes.
Now you'll have to get whatever cigarettes you want from other smokers. This will make smoking an even more conscious act than asking for a light. We're not trying to embarrass you out of smoking, just to give you a better chance of practicing the kind of self-control you're going to need tomorrow, because . . .

Tomorrow you'll quit smoking for 24 hours.
That's right. Tomorrow you're going to stop smoking for twenty-four hours, and today you should psych yourself up for the event. Call your friends. Tell them—your nonsmoking or ex-smoker friends—that you're quitting. They'll give you lots of encouragement, but the real reason for doing this is to declare your intentions and commit yourself more fully.

Clean your ashtrays at the end of the day.
Put the butts in a glass jar if you can find one, so you can look at them and take off the lid and take a sniff tomorrow if you're tempted to smoke.

Look in the mirror and put a big smile on your face!
He who laughs last laughs best, and now that you've survived these first five days and you're committed to quitting for the next twenty-four hours, you deserve a few laughs.

Keep up the breathing exercises.
Keep up with your walks or other aerobic exercise.

DAY 6

Don't smoke for 24 hours.
If you can get through this day, the next will be easier, and easier, and easier, until after a while the urge to smoke will leave you and you'll wonder why you didn't quit years ago.

The battle isn't over yet, though, and you should be very wary today. Avoid the patterns that you've discovered connect you to the smoking habit. Especially avoid alcohol, because alcohol lowers your resistance to temptation, and you'll need all the willpower you can muster today.

Avoid all situations that you normally associate with smoking. You know what they are.

If you're tempted to have a cigarette, don't do it. Do something else. Try a breathing exercise, or a stick of gum, or take a walk around the block.

Call your friends to report on your progress.
Remember, call only nonsmokers. Smoking friends may pooh-pooh your accomplishment with cracks about how many times they've quit. Your smoking friends will not be supportive; they may in fact be a trifle resentful of your success and feel it is a reflection on their own willpower if you rid yourself of a dependency they haven't escaped.

So call your nonsmoking friends. Ex-smokers will be particularly appreciative and supportive, because they've been through it too. They may even have some helpful suggestions about how to resist the temptation to start smoking again.

The following tips will help you maintain your nonsmoking habit:
- Make up a short list of luxuries you have wanted or items you would like to purchase as a gift for someone. Next to each item write down the cost in terms of packs of cigarettes. Use a special piggy bank for the money you don't spend on cigarettes, or start a Christmas Club account at your bank.
- Try going to bed early and rising a half-hour earlier than usual to avoid hurrying through breakfast and rushing to work.
- Keep your hands occupied. Try playing a musical instrument, knitting or fiddling with hand puzzles.
- Take a shower. You cannot smoke in the shower.
- If you have a sudden craving for a cigarette, take ten deep breaths, holding the last breath while you strike a match. Exhale slowly, blowing out the match. Pretend the match was a cigarette by crushing it

out in an ashtray. Now immediately get busy on some work or activity.

- After you quit, start using your lungs. Increase your activities and try a new sport, say paddle tennis, or handball, or some form of moderate exercise, such as short walks or a bicycle ride before or after a meal.
- If you gain weight because you miss smoking, wait until you get over the wish to smoke before you diet. Dieting is easier then.
- When you feel irritable or tense, shut your eyes and count backward from ten to zero as you imagine yourself descending a flight of stairs, or imagine you are looking at the horizon as the sun sets in the west.
- Stock up on light reading materials, crossword puzzles and vacation brochures you can read during your coffee breaks.
- Frequent places in which you can't smoke, such as libraries, buses, theaters, swimming pools, department stores—or just go to bed during the first weeks you are off cigarettes.

Keep up the breathing exercises. Take your walk.
Maintaining the nonsmoking habit can be as hard as quitting for some people. You'll find lots of helpful suggestions here that have been tried successfully by other ex-smokers. They won't all work for you, but if you find one or two that will help you through those times of stress or depression when you really wish you had a cigarette, they will have served you well.

DAY 7

Remember, if you got through one day you can get through another.
This day will be easier than yesterday. Most smokers don't believe they can really get through a whole day without smoking. You've done it! Doing it again should be easier.

But don't let down your guard! Cockiness is the worst enemy of the ex-smoker. Keep planning. Continue consciously to stay away from coffee and drinks and any other situations you associate with smoking.

Keep busy. Keep active. Don't give yourself a chance to think about smoking.

Keep exercising.
Your lungs should feel cleaner already. Truly. You may cough more than usual, but that's the lungs' cleansing mechanism at work.

All trace of cigarette taste will have disappeared from your mouth by now. Breathe deeply and enjoy that good fresh air. Take a walk. (We hope it isn't raining or snowing.) If it's raining, stick your head out the door and smell the rain. Smell some fresh flowers, or an apple or an orange.

Save the money you're not spending on cigarettes.
Put the price of the cigarettes you used to smoke in some safe place. Add to it every day, and when you've saved your cigarette money for a few weeks, buy yourself a present. If you save that money for a year, you'll probably actually be able to take a vacation trip that you wouldn't otherwise have taken.

If you broke down and had a cigarette yesterday, don't give up.
Pick yourself up, dust yourself off and stay away from cigarettes today. If you're really having difficulty, go back to day 4 and work your way on from there.

There's no disgrace in failing. Review what worked for you and think about what didn't. But don't quit quitting. Get going again.

DAY 8

Congratulate yourself!
You've been off cigarettes for two days! Stick with it. And welcome to the honorable and growing order of ex-smokers.

You've just saved yourself several hundred dollars a year in very non-deductible expenses. (Think of how much you had to earn before taxes to pay for your smoking habit. Then gloat.)

And statistics show that you've probably added about five years to your life span, and you've added immeasurably to your enjoyment of life.

Focus on your unexpected benefits.
You may have started to experience unexpected benefits of smoking, such as an increase in your self-esteem, or you may have become increasingly assertive. These are examples of serendipity, the ripple effect or unexpected benefits.

Try to handle withdrawal symptoms.
Some but not all new ex-smokers experience withdrawal symptoms. These include:

- craving
- headache
- tension
- gastrointestinal disturbances
- irritability
- anxiety reactions
- restlessness
- difficulty concentrating
- lightheadedness or dizziness
- coughing

Most of these symptoms are really symptoms of recovery, making you feel worse rather than better. Just be patient; most of them disappear within two and a half weeks. It is important for you to understand that the unpleasant aftereffects of quitting are only temporary and signal the beginning of a healthier life.

If your craving comes on strong, touch your toes ten times, call a friend, try low-calorie snacks or do the deep-breathing exercises you learned. For the other symptoms, try a muscle relaxation exercise from chapter 6 or go for a brisk walk.

Check your ashtray.
Doesn't it look good! No cigarette butts.

Review the major benefits of stopping smoking from day 2.

DAYS 9–14

Continue the good work.
You're doing great. If you've had a bad time and slipped once or twice, don't worry about it. Forge ahead! Study your Smoking Record. This is a consciousness reinforcement procedure. You are taking control of your life.

Participate in a daily exercise program.
If you are not already doing one of the aerobic exercise programs in chapter 2, select one and perform the exercises every day. The feeling of health and vigor afforded by exercise is a strong deterrent against smoking.

Learn the various exercises in chapter 6 to reduce stress.

The amount of concentration that is required to remember not to smoke and to resist the multiple temptations to smoke is stressful. You must engage in the breathing, muscle relaxation and meditation exercises in chapter 6 on a regular basis without fail. It is necessary to learn them extremely well and practice them several times each day so that you can relax your body with a minimum of effort. Also practice the fantasy exercise and muscle relaxation exercise described on pages 121 and 122 several times a day so that they can be done with a minimum of effort.

Try various ways to keep your hands busy.

It is important to keep your hands occupied so that you won't reach for a cigarette. Some ways to do this at home include:

- Do crossword puzzles.
- Do needlework.
- Garden.
- Write letters.
- Play Ping-Pong.
- Do household chores.
- Learn to use a home computer.
- Do crafts.
- Wash your car.
- Trim your nails.

Think of other long-term benefits of stopping smoking.

In addition to those major benefits of stopping smoking listed on day 1, more and more benefits will be realized:

1. Your lung capacity will increase.
2. If you have smoker's cough, it will disappear.
3. Your risk of contracting various cancers will decrease progressively until you have no more risk than a person who never smoked.

Develop new habits to counter fatigue and weight gain.

1. Get enough rest so that you are at your best physically and mentally.
2. Eat five or six small meals instead of two or three big ones.
3. Eat foods as given in chapter 3.
4. Drink a lot of the right fluids, such as water to increase your circulation and stimulate digestion, skim milk to soothe your nerves and avoid fatigue, citrus or tomato juice to give you a quick energy boost.

5. *Learn the meditation method in chapter 6.* Practice it at the same time each day for 20 minutes (see p. 120), or turn to page 121 for a relaxation fantasy.

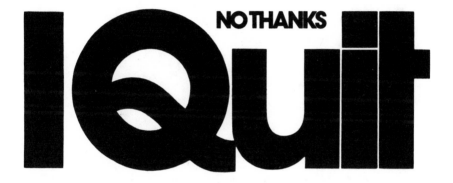

The 14-Day Heart-Saving

Blood Pressure

Control Plan

> *Progress comes from the intelligent use of experi-*
> *ence.*
> —Elbert Hubbard

WHAT IS HIGH BLOOD PRESSURE?

Your blood pressure consists of two numbers—a high one and a low one (e.g., 140/90). The high number, called the *systolic blood pressure*, is the highest pressure or force of the blood against the walls of the arteries during the time the heart is contracting to pump blood into the circulation. The lower number is the *diastolic blood pressure*. It is the lowest pressure against the walls of the arteries in between beats when the heart is at rest. If the systolic blood pressure is below 140 and the diastolic blood pressure is below 90, blood pressure is considered normal. Occasionally the blood pressure will rise above these values with exercise, anxiety, stress or even when the blood pressure cuff is attached to a person's arm. This does not constitute high blood pressure unless the pressure remains above these values while the person is at rest.

The Effect of High Blood Pressure on the Heart

Increased blood pressure forces the heart to work harder, causing it gradually to enlarge. It may eventually precipitate heart failure. Sustained high blood pressure may have a deteriorating effect on the blood vessels, thereby accelerating the atherosclerotic process. Moreover, some believe that if a person has a high level of cholesterol and fats in the blood, an elevated blood pressure may drive these substances into the arterial wall at a faster rate than normal. Therefore a person with normal or subnormal blood pressure may possibly tolerate a higher fat and cholesterol level than one with high blood pressure. Hypertension also takes its toll on the small blood vessels of the kidneys, causing them to thicken progressively, thereby reducing the blood flow and eventually leading to kidney failure. The blood vessels of the brain are also susceptible to high blood pressure, leading to strokes.

FACTORS AFFECTING BLOOD PRESSURE

Heredity

We don't know for sure whether blood pressure levels are genetically determined, but what we do know is that high blood pressure runs in families. People whose parents have high blood pressure are more likely to develop it than those whose parents do not have the disease. Some doctors say the association is environmental, based entirely on nutritional and other habits developed in the home. Others think it's due to a genetic inability to handle salt. Still others believe that it is a combination of genetic factors influenced by environmental factors.

Salt and High Blood Pressure

Most experts agree that there is a definite link between salt and high blood pressure. Therefore, you must make every effort to reduce the salt content of your food. It is also of major importance that you form the habit of reading labels and learn how to calculate the sodium content of your foods. (Refer to Mastering Good Eating Habits, p. 67.)

Exercise

In a study published in 1984 in the *Journal of the American Medical Association* that involved 6,039 men and women ages twenty to sixty-five years of age who were followed for one to twelve years, it was found that those who were physically fit were less likely to develop high blood pressure than those with low fitness levels.

Weight Reduction

Weight reduction has long been associated with a fall in blood pressure for overweight people. Yet many physicians treat their overweight patients with medications without doing anything about their weight. In many instances weight reduction alone may be sufficient to normalize a person's blood pressure. Therefore, the first step to successfully lowering your blood pressure is weight reduction.

Dietary Modification

A study published in 1983 that was conducted in England using a low-fat, high-fiber, low-sodium, reduced-calorie diet resulted in a significant reductin of blood pressure. The 14-Day Heart-Saving Menu Plan provided in chapter 3 will assure a low-fat, high-fiber, low-sodium diet. This dietary plan requires a gradual change in life-style, but the rewards are great.

Cigarette Smoking and High Blood Pressure

The nicotine in cigarettes constricts blood vessels, causing the blood pressure to rise. It also increases heart rate by as much as 33 beats a minute. Although the rise may not be very high in all cases, it still contributes to the overall picture. A cigarette smoker with high blood pressure has a greatly increased risk of developing cardiovascular disease. The Framingham study revealed that forty-year-old male smokers with high blood pressure were three and a half times more likely to develop cardiovascular disease than were forty-year-old males without these risks.

Drugs to Lower Blood Pressure

There is currently a large arsenal of drugs available to control high blood pressure that are used singly or in combination. Unfortunately most of these drugs may cause side effects that are numerous and vary according to the drug used. This is compounded by combination therapy, which uses two or more drugs at the same time. One drug manufacturer lists over eighty side effects on the package instructions that range from simple nausea to serious blood disorders. Recent reports on high blood pressure therapy that dealt a nasty blow to the medical community was the finding that the diuretic drugs, the beta blockers and perhaps other blood pressure drugs may significantly raise the total cholesterol, bad cholesterol and triglycerides and lower the good cholesterol in many individuals. This raises the suspicion that medical treatment with these drugs might actually augment coronary disease instead of preventing it. However, no long-term studies demonstrating such an effect have been reported. Regardless, *blood-pressure-lowering drugs should be avoided whenever possible, and when drugs have to be used, the lowest dose possible should be given.* Moreover, if diuretics and beta blockers are used, the total cholesterol, the good cholesterol and the triglyceride blood levels should be taken before and after treatment to determine if they are significantly affected by the medication.

Lowering Blood Pressure Without Drugs

Several scientific investigations have shown that high blood pressure can be significantly lowered without drugs. One notable study conducted in 1980 by the Chicago Coronary Prevention Evaluation Program did just that. The blood pressures of 115 mildly hypertensive men were reduced to normal without drugs after they adopted an improved life-style with regard to eating, exercising and smoking habits. Interestingly, following the "Controversies in Cardiology" Debates at the 33rd Annual Scientific Session of the American College of Cardiology at Dallas in 1984, 291 cardiologists who attended indicated on a questionnaire that they were against using pharmacologic drugs for mild high blood pressure, as opposed to 232 who were for it and 70 who were undecided.

THE 14-DAY HEART-SAVING BLOOD PRESSURE-LOWERING PLAN

The 14-Day Heart-Saving Blood Pressure-Lowering Plan contains all the basic principles for successfully lowering high blood pressure. These include:

1. reducing your weight to normal
2. restricting your sodium intake
3. controlling stress
4. exercising regularly
5. quitting smoking
6. eating a low-fat, high-fiber, low-sodium, calorie-restricted diet
7. avoiding oral contraceptives

A word of caution: If you are presently on high blood pressure medication, do not stop taking it without first checking with your doctor. The best approach in this situation is to inform your physician of your intentions to lower your blood pressure so that your progress can be checked periodically. You might have to stay on the drugs, reducing them gradually as you lower your blood pressure. If you find that your pressure is moderately to severely high and you are not on medication, you should also check with your physician, who may begin drug treatment while you are on the program. If your blood pressure elevation is mild, you could begin the program while you monitor your own progress. However, it would be prudent to first have a medical checkup to rule out the small percentage of discoverable causes of high blood pressure. If you are unsuccessful in lowering your pressure using this program, you must consult your physician.

DAY 1

Purchase a blood pressure unit.
Blood pressure units vary in price from about $20 to several hundred dollars and can be purchased at drugstores, surgical supply houses, department stores, mail-order and catalog houses or through your doctor. I would recommend that you purchase an outfit complete with stethoscope in the price range of $25 to $30. Units are available that have a stethoscope already attached, so that you can take your own blood pressure completely alone. Beware of the home electronic blood pressure apparatus that eliminates the need for a stethoscope by having a transducer for sensing the Korotov sounds built into the cuff. When the air is released, a beeping sound and/or flashing light begins with the systolic pressure and stops with the diastolic pressure. It is great in principle and simple to use, but there is one catch—accuracy! These units can be unreliable, particularly in the diastolic pressure range.

Learn to take your own blood pressure.
The instrument used to take your blood pressure is called a *sphygmomanometer* and consists of an inflatable cuff to wrap around the arm, a bulb to inflate the cuff and a gauge to read the blood pressure (see diagram). A stethoscope is included to listen to the sounds that occur in the artery (Korotov sounds) while taking the blood pressure.

Wrap the inflatable cuff snugly around your upper arm just above the elbow, as depicted in the illustration. A symbol (arrow, circle, dot, etc.) is generally marked on the cuff designating the exact spot on the cuff that must be aligned with the artery (brachial artery). This artery runs along

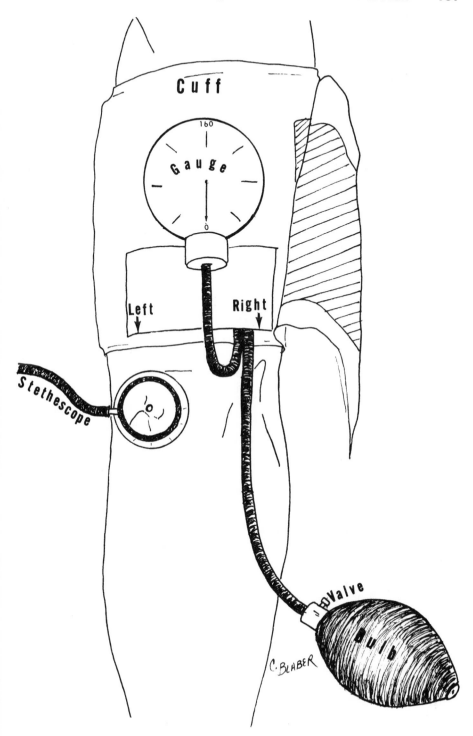

the inside of the forearm. Place the diaphragm or bell of the stethoscope over the artery just below the symbol on the cuff. Have someone hold the stethoscope in place for you. Close the valve on the bulb by turning the knob clockwise, and inflate the cuff to a high reading on the gauge (about 180). Open the valve slightly in a counterclockwise direction to release the air very slowly while listening with the stethoscope for the first discernible Korotov sounds. Record the reading on the gauge exactly at the time the sounds are first heard. This is the systolic pressure. Continue releasing the air until you no longer hear the sounds. The pressure reading on the gauge when the sounds first disappear is the diastolic pressure.

The procedure may vary slightly according to the design of the instrument, so consult the instructions that accompany it. The best way to learn to use one is to have your doctor, a nurse or a paramedic teach you.

DAY 2

If you are overweight, study the 14-Day Low-Fat Low-Cholesterol Weight-Reduction Plan today (see Appendix A) and set up a program to lose 2 pounds each week. It is important that you adhere strictly to the program.

Restrict your salt intake, particularly if your blood pressure is affected by it. The best way to determine if your blood pressure is salt-related is to check your blood pressure before and after consuming a salt-rich diet for a week or two. It would be prudent to let your physician determine this for you, as she or he is skilled in making this type of judgment.

Starting today, make it a habit to avoid using the salt shaker. Perhaps paint a skull and crossbones with the word *poison* on it.

Read the food labels of everything you eat for sources of sodium you might not think of. Many food seasonings and staples are high in sodium. Monosodium glutamate or MSG (a flavor enhancer), sodium saccharin (a sweetener), sodium caseinate (a thickener and binder), sodium phosphates (emulsifiers, stabilizers and buffers), sodium benzoate and sodium nitrate (preservatives) are all prime examples. Baking powder and baking soda are sodium compounds, and some canned and frozen fruits and most canned whole tomatoes are dipped in sodium hydroxide for easy peeling. Other hidden sources of sodium include the use of sodium citrate to buffer some canned and bottled citrus drinks and the use of sodium ion exchange to reduce sediment in some wines. Avoid the use of antacids containing sodium compounds. There are several good ones without sodium.

Check the labels on your frozen foods as well. Don't assume they don't have added salt. Frozen vegetables are usually processed without adding salt, but starchy vegetables including lima beans and peas are frequently sorted in salt solution prior to freezing. Although frozen fruits are not usually processed with added salt, some manufacturers add small amounts of salt to prevent darkening as well as to enhance the flavor of applesauce.

Check the sodium content of your water supply with your water company, because there is a marked variation throughout the country. Remember, the production and bottling of soft drinks and beer would also be affected according to the water source utilized.

DAY 3

Continue restricting salt. Wash the salt off various foods. Many food products such as water-packed tuna and other canned goods can be washed briefly under running water. This removes a large amount of the salt.

Starting today, avoid the following high-sodium foods (a complete list of food items with their sodium content is given in the Appendix).

salt	salt pork
pretzels	fast foods in general
potato chips	sardines
salted peanuts	baking soda and powder
catsup	canned foods where sodium value is not given
frankfurters	cake mixes
smoked meats	soy sauce
smoked fish	salted french fries
pickles and pickled	
foods	mustard
anchovies	celery salt
garlic salt	antacids with sodium
onion salt	salted nuts
Worcestershire	
sauce	

DAY 4

Explore new ways to flavor food. Today go out and buy a salt substitute. Stock up on simple replacements such as lemon juice, vinegar, onion, wines and pepper. The following list, recommended by the Food Market Institutes, shows herbs and herb mixtures and the various dishes they enhance. They can be made up and stored. Completely crush the herbs in order to extract their full flavor. Recently dried herbs are more flavorful than those that are stored for long periods.

anise seed: fruit, fruit salads, cakes, cookies, breads and fish

basil: pork chops or roast, meat loaf and rice

bay leaf: soups, chowders, fish, pot roast and marinades

chili powder: ground beef, noodles or rice, pot roast, barbecue sauce, tomatoes and dips

cumin: meat loaf, hamburger, pot roast, stews, lentil and pea soups, tomato sauce, egg dishes, rice, salad dressing and potato salad

dill weed: green vegetables, cooked noodles, fish, chicken, breads and eggs

dry mustard: salad dressings, meat, poultry and vegetables

fennel seed: fish, seafood, artichokes, cauliflower, broccoli, Brussels sprouts, potatoes, baked goods, tomato sauce and spaghetti

garlic: green salads, green beans, tomatoes, eggplant, salad dressing, beef, lamb, veal, variety meat, fish and seafood

nutmeg: mixed vegetables, ground beef, chicken, tuna and baked goods

oregano: egg salad, green beans, tomatoes, pasta sauces, vegetable soup, stuffings, pork, lamb, chicken and fish

paprika: beef, pork, veal, lamb, fish, poultry, potatoes and other white vegetables

rosemary: lamb, poultry, veal, beef, pork, fish, soups, stews, marinades, potatoes, cauliflower, fruits and breads

saffron: baked goods, chicken, seafood, rice, soups and international dishes

sage: sauces, soups, chowders, poultry, fish, beef, pork, veal, marinades, lima beans, onions, eggplant, tomatoes and potatoes

tarragon: casseroles, marinades, pot roast, veal, lamb, poultry, fish, seafood, egg dishes and green salads

thyme: beef, poultry, fish and vegetables

Stir-Fry Spice

1 teaspoon fresh grated lemon peel
¼ teaspoon crushed anise seed
¼ teaspoon crushed fennel seed
¼ teaspoon ground cinnamon
¼ teaspoon ground cloves
¼ teaspoon ground ginger

Combine all ingredients. Refrigerate in a covered container. To use, sprinkle as desired over poultry or meat stir-fry dishes. Makes about 2 teaspoons.

One-half teaspoon equal 1 milligram sodium, 2 calories.

Herb Shaker
½ teaspoon cayenne pepper
1 tablespoon garlic powder
1 teaspoon each of ground basil, marjoram, thyme, parsley, savory and mace
1 teaspoon onion powder
1 teaspoon black pepper
1 teaspoon sage

Combine ingredients and place in a salt shaker.

Lemon-Herb Seasoning
Grated peel of one lemon
2 tablespoons ground cinnamon
1 tablespoon ground mace
1 tablespoon dried crushed basil leaves
1 tablespoon dried crushed thyme leaves
1 tablespoon dried crushed rosemary leaves
2 teaspoons paprika
1 teaspoon salt substitute
1 teaspoon pepper
1 teaspoon ground cloves
½ teaspoon ground nutmeg
½ teaspoon ground allspice

Combine all ingredients. Refrigerate in a covered container. To use, sprinkle as desired over meat, poultry or fish before broiling or baking. Makes about ½ cup.

One teaspoon equals 47 milligrams sodium, 5 calories.

DAY 5

Begin a stress-reduction program.
The 14-Day Heart-Saving Stress Control Plan in chapter 6 teaches you how to control stress using behavior modification techniques, stress reduction methods, stress relaxation methods and exercise, all of which are incorporated into a person's daily activities. The meditation method and muscle relaxation techniques in particular have been very successful in lowering high blood pressure. Mild cases of high blood pressure can frequently be controlled without drugs if these methods are used faithfully. In practically all cases of high blood pressure, less medication is required. The meditation method is a simple technique that is easy to learn, simple to use and can easily be adapted to your own life-style. Incorporate two periods of ten to fifteen minutes each into your schedule each day, and

practice this technique every day without fail. Transcendental meditation is also a very effective technique but requires a training program given by special teachers. The muscle relaxation techniques given in chapter 6 should be practiced daily, as they are also effective in lowering the blood pressure by counteracting stress.

1. Determine two 10- to 15-minute periods each day during which you would be least apt to be disturbed, and incorporate these times into your daily schedule.
2. Select a quiet area of your home that is conducive to relaxation.
3. Follow the Meditation procedure on page 120.
4. During the day, practice one or more of the muscle relaxation techniques described in chapter 6.

DAY 6

If you haven't already, begin a regular exercise program today. Aerobic exercises are also quite effective in lowering high blood pressure, but they must be done regularly. The 14-Day Heart-Saving Exercise Plan in chapter 2 is designed to help you select an exercise program that is best for you and provides you with a series of aerobic exercise programs that are excellent for this purpose. Select a program according to your personal requirements and incorporate it into your daily schedule. It is very important that you start the 14-Day Heart-Saving Exercise Plan in chapter 2 right from the very beginning of the chapter, including the Health Check Quiz.

DAY 7

Study the 14-Day Heart-Saving Diet Plan in chapter 3 today. Then proceed to change your dietary life-style gradually according to the format in chapter 10.

If you are a smoker, study the 14-Day Heart-Saving Quit-Smoking Plan in chapter 4. Set a date on your calendar to begin this two-week program and adhere to it rigorously.

DAYS 8–14

1. Continue with your weight reduction program. Make it a practice to weigh yourself once each week.
2. Restrict the salt in your diet on a permanent basis if your blood

pressure is affected by salt. Review the recommendations given on day 3.

3. Continue learning the principles of the 14-Day Heart-Saving Menu Plan given in chapter 3 and the vitamin and mineral recommendations given in chapter 7 and begin putting them to use.
4. Do your meditation method at the same time every day.
5. Put the stress reduction techniques you learned in chapter 6 to work on a daily basis to cope with the stressful events of the day.
6. Exercise regularly.
7. Avoid oral contraceptives. Oral contraceptives have been shown to raise blood pressure significantly. Therefore, they should be avoided whenever possible. Consult with your physician for advice before stopping use of them.

YOUR EXERCISE PRESCRIPTION FOR LOWER BLOOD PRESSURE

Strict adherence to these recommendations in most instances will either reduce your blood pressure to normal without drugs or bring it to a lower level, requring either a smaller dose of drugs or a milder, less toxic drug. So you have every reason to start your 14-Day Blood Pressure Control Plan today.

Chapter Six

The 14-Day Heart-Saving

Stress Control Plan

*Future shock . . . the shattering stress and disori-
entation that we induce in individuals by subject-
ing them to too much in too short a time.*
                                          —Alvin Toffler

The 14-Day Heart-Saving Stress Control Plan is designed to combat the
many facets of stress with which we so often come into contact.

This plan begins by evaluating your stress level according to a simple
test. This is a highly reliable way to predict your changes of getting sick
from stress. This test is based on the studies of Drs. Thomas Holmes and
Richard Rahe, who correlated forty-three important life-event items that
commonly occurred before the onset of illness, such as the death of a
spouse, trouble with one's boss, being fired, changing jobs, getting di-
vorced and so on. They found that the higher one's stress score, the
greater one's chance of experiencing an illness over the next two years.

PREVENTIVE MEASURES
Dr. Holmes also compiled the following suggestions for using the stress
test to stay healthy. Try to follow them.

1. Become familiar with the life events and the amount of change they
   require.
2. Put the scale where you and the family can see it several times a
   day.

3. Practice so that you can recognize when a life event happens.
4. Think about the meaning of the event for you and try to identify some of the feelings you experience.
5. Think about the different ways you might best adjust to the event.
6. Take your time in arriving at decisions.
7. If possible, anticipate life changes and plan for them well in advance.
8. Pace yourself. It can be done even if you are in a hurry.
9. Look at the accomplishment of a task as part of daily living and avoid viewing such an achievement as a stopping point or a time for letting down.
10. Remember, the more change you have, the more likely you are to get sick. Of those people with 300 or more Life Change Units for the past year, almost 80% get sick in the near future; with 150 to 299 Life Change Units, about 50% get sick in the near future; and with less than 150 Life Change Units, only about 30% get sick in the near future. So the higher your Life Change Score, the harder you must work to stay well.

The Social Readjustment Rating Scale

	Life Event	Mean Value
1.	Death of spouse	100
2.	Divorce	73
3.	Marital separation from mate	65
4.	Detention in jail or other institution	63
5.	Death of a close family member	63
6.	Major personal injury or illness	53
7.	Marriage	50
8.	Being fired at work	47
9.	Marital reconciliation with mate	45
10.	Retirement from work	45
11.	Major change in the health or behavior of a family member	44
12.	Pregnancy	40
13.	Sexual difficulties	39
14.	Gaining a new family member (e.g., through birth, adoption, oldster moving in, etc.)	39
15.	Major business readjustment (e.g., merger, reorganization, bankruptcy, etc.)	39
16.	Major change in financial state (e.g., a lot worse off or a lot better off than usual)	38
17.	Death of a close friend	37
18.	Changing to a different line of work	36

The Social Readjustment Rating Scale (cont.)

Life Event	Mean Value
19. Major change in the number of arguments with spouse (e.g., either a lot more or a lot less than usual regarding child-rearing, personal habits, etc.)	35
20. Taking out a mortgage or loan for a major purchase (e.g., for a home, business, etc.)	31
21. Foreclosure on a mortgage or loan	30
22. Major change in responsibilities at work (e.g., promotion, demotion, lateral transfer)	29
23. Son or daughter leaving home (e.g., marriage, attending college, etc.)	29
24. Trouble with in-laws	29
25. Outstanding personal achievement	28
26. Wife beginning or ceasing work outside the home	26
27. Beginning or ceasing formal schooling	26
28. Major change in living conditions (e.g., building a new home, remodeling, deterioration of home or neighborhood)	25
29. Revision of personal habits (dress, manners, associations, etc.)	24
30. Trouble with the boss	23
31. Major change in working hours or conditions	20
32. Change in residence	20
33. Changing to a new school	20
34. Major change in usual type and/or amount of recreation	19
35. Major change in church activities (e.g., a lot more or a lot less than usual)	19
36. Major change in social activities (e.g., clubs, dancing, movies, visiting, etc.)	18
37. Taking out a mortgage or loan for a lesser purchase (e.g., for a car, TV, freezer, etc.)	17
38. Major change in sleeping habits (a lot more or a lot less sleep, or change in part of day when asleep)	16
39. Major change in number of family get-togethers (e.g., a lot more or a lot less than usual)	15
40. Major change in eating habits (a lot more or a lot less food intake, or very different meal hours or surroundings)	15
41. Vacation	13
42. Christmas	12
43. Minor violations of the law (e.g., traffic tickets, jaywalking, disturbing the peace, etc.)	11

Reprinted with permission from Holmes, T. H, and Rahe, R. H., "The Social Readjustment Rating Scale," Journal of Psychosomatic Research 11: 213–218, 1967, and Pergamon Press, Ltd.

BEHAVIORAL PROFILE QUESTIONNAIRE

The following questionnaire is used to determine if you have a type A or type B personality and to what extreme. It is the extreme A people who have the greatest risk of having a heart attack. This profile also identifies those characteristics that need changing.

Place a check after each of the following questions if the answer is yes.

1. Are you aggressive?
2. Are you competitive?
3. Is it important that you win?
4. Do you become hostile if things don't go your way?
5. Are you easily annoyed?
6. Are you driven to make money, to be successful or to climb to the top?
7. Do you frequently tense your facial muscles?
8. Are you easily irritated by other drivers?
9. Do you get tense and ready to fight when another motorist makes a remark to you?
10. Do you become irritated when waiting on lines at the bank or in a store or at the station, etc.?
11. Are you easily provoked to anger?
12. Do you frequently shake your knee rapidly or tap on a counter or tabletop while waiting or during meetings?
13. Do you walk fast to your various destinations?
14. Do you drive fast to your various destinations?
15. Do you have difficulty delegating tasks?
16. Do you pound the table during discussions?
17. Do you schedule many activities into less time?
18. Do you have difficulty relaxing when away from the job?
19. Do you eat fast?
20. Do you speak fast?
21. Do you constantly bring work home from the job?
22. Do you have difficulty relaxing when watching TV, when out to dinner, when on vacation?
23. Do you feel driven to get a job done?
24. Do you try to do more and more in less time?
25. Do you constantly feel threatened?

If you check less than five items, you probably are not a type A; if you check more than five, you probably are a type A; if you check more than ten, you probably are an extreme type A. If you fit the type A profile, then the stress control plan is particularly important for you to follow.

BEGINNING THE 14-DAY HEART-SAVING STRESS CONTROL PLAN

Combatting stress is accomplished through behavior modification techniques, stress reduction methods, relaxation methods and exercise, all of which are incorporated into a person's daily activities.

To manage stress successfully, it is important to know the ways it is experienced and what the hazards of chronic stress are. Stress comes from different sources. Every aspect of a person's environment is fraught with stress. There are job tensions, home and social pressures, weather influences, economic pressures, ego threats, security threats, noise levels, time requirements and many more. These are *environmental stresses*. Some stresses result from worry and lead to agitation, tension, fear and hypochondria; these are *mental stresses*. Still other stresses are the consequences of natural attrition of the body from aging, illness, nutritional disturbances, biochemical imbalances, medications and physical inactivity. These are *bodily* or *physiological stresses*.

Now let's learn how to reduce stress by using the 14-Day Heart-Saving Stress Control Plan.

DAY 1

1. Prepare a Stress Notebook to demonstrate to yourself just how the specific stressful events you encounter actually precipitate specific symptoms and permit you to select the most effective methods for counteracting specific stressful events.

   Title the first page "Stressful Situations," and prepare a list of the stressful situations you usually encounter under the subtitles "To and From Work," "At Work," "At Home" and "During Social Activities." Now add the information you checked on the Social Readjustment Rating Scale to this list. Make another list of the behavioral characteristics that you propose to change, such as aggression, hostility, impatience, overwork and so on. Consult your Behavioral Profile for any additional characteristics and add them to the list.

   Now, prepare a sheet with the title "Daily Stress Experiences." Place the following headings across the top of the sheet: "Time," "Stress Experience," "Feeling" and "Action Taken." This sheet must be filled out every day with your stress experiences and the actions you took to counteract them. This must be done from the time you awaken in the morning until you go to bed at night. The first few lines might look like those in the following chart. At the beginning of the program, very little will be written under "Action Taken," but this will increase as you progress in the program.

Daily Stress Experiences

Time	Experience	Feeling	Action Taken
10 A.M.	waiting in line at the bank	aggravation	read magazine
1 P.M.	admonished by boss	tense	muscle relaxation
5 P.M.	remark by motorist	angry	poem recitation and breathing exercise
8 P.M.	thoughts about a trip contemplated next month	fear	thought-breaking procedure

2. Starting today and for each day of your 14-day program, do not sit down to a large meal immediately at the end of your workday. Begin to unwind, leaving the problems of the day at the job. The pressures of the job, with its aggravation, deadlines, arguments, abuse from superiors, auto troubles on the way home and so on, when added to a large evening meal, can be the last straw that results in a heart attack. It is important to wait about an hour before eating. Take a warm, *not hot*, shower, get into comfortable clothing, put on some relaxing music and enjoy a cup of tea, a cocktail, a glass of wine or a cold beer. (This may even avoid an argument at home as to why dinner may not have been ready.)

3. Try to relax after work. Today, adopt a new rule of not taking your work home. Instead, go in early or leave a little later. And starting today, if you commute to work alone, listen to music on your car radio or cassette player so that you can relax. Or use this time to listen to learning cassettes, which are available on most subjects: vocabulary building, foreign languages, music appreciation, investments, health and so on. These aids are a great help in getting your mind off the events experienced during the day.

4. Exercise for 15 to 20 minutes every day. Follow the instructions given in the 14-Day Heart-Saving Exercise Plan (chapter 2) in selecting a program suited to your needs. Aerobic exercise is a great way to eliminate stress and provide for more relaxed sleep patterns. It also affords a high level of relaxation and decreases high blood pressure.

5. You might also learn the following meditation method and perform it every day for 20 minutes. This method should be done at the same time each day, preferably when you are least apt to be disturbed and when it is quiet.

   Meditation methods afford a high level of relaxation and are a tremendous aid in reducing all types of stress, decreasing high blood pressure and relieving muscle tension. They also promote restful sleep.

For centuries people have found that deep within our bodies is an ability to relax totally, just as the fight-or-flight reaction stimulates the entire body to react to danger. The opposite effect of relaxation is innate in every one of us. Practitioners of transcendental meditation and yoga have discovered this and put it to great use, but unfortunately the various procedures for attaining a relaxation state were placed in the realm of mysticism until Dr. Herbert Benson, a cardiologist at Boston's Beth Israel Hospital and a professor at Harvard Medical School, showed that he could simplify the technique of transcendental meditation by eliminating some of the mysticism and putting it to work in a very practical manner. His studies revealed significant decreases in blood pressure and reduction of certain rhythm abnormalities of the heart.

Meditation Method

a. Two hours or more after eating, sit quietly and comfortably in a chair and close your eyes.
b. Concentrate on relaxing all your muscles, beginning at the feet and working up gradually to the legs, torso, arms and neck and face.
c. Think of the word *one* or a word or phrase that you have a personal belief in, such as a religious word or phrase. Then begin to breathe through your nose, reciting this word silently to yourself each time you breathe out while keeping the word or phrase in your mind. (Some people have excellent results using a pet word or prayer instead of using the word *one*. An example is the religious phrase "Oh Lord have mercy," "alleluia" or ""Jesus I love you." Benson refers to a combination of the relaxation method with a person's belief system as the faith factor).

Keep repeating the word or phrase you selected over and over each time you breathe out, while concentrating on nothing. Ignore any distracting thoughts and let them float into your head and out again. This should be done for about 15 to 20 minutes, without using an alarm clock, but place a clock or watch where it can easily be checked. It is important to get into the habit of doing this at exactly the same time every day.

Perform the following fantasy meditation exercise as an alternate to the meditation method. It is very soothing and relieves deep tension.

Fantasy Meditation Exercise

Sit down for this exercise. Make yourself completely comfortable, and close your eyes. Inhale deeply and exhale slowly. Think only of letting your body relax like a rag doll.

Now count from one to ten as follows. When you get to ten, you will be in a state of extremely deep relaxation. One: you are more and more relaxed. Two: the room is fading away. Three: all your tension is disappearing. Four: you feel very quiet. Five: these feelings become deeper and deeper. Six: relax even more. Seven: your tension is completely gone. Eight: the nerves and muscles of your body now want only to rest. Nine: you are totally relaxed.

Now in this very relaxed state, picture yourself walking quietly and slowly down a path by a mountain meadow, down by a quiet, still lake. It is early morning and the sun is shining warmly and air is cool and sweet. You can smell the sweet pines and the grass, and occasionally a fish jumps in the lake; the lake is deep, deep blue and very still. You sit down slowly in the grass at the edge of the lake and relax. A gentle breeze rustles the grass very softly, and you look up at the blue sky and there are white clouds floating past.

You lie and watch the clouds, and then you begin to float up to the clouds. You are able to walk around on the clouds, and it is fun. It is warm, and the air is clean and fresh, and the sky is blue and the clouds are soft and white and springy. You feel the warm sun, and as you breathe in, you feel your whole body fill with the fresh, clear air, and you are extremely relaxed.

Now you begin to wake up slowly, and you are here, seated comfortably, and you still feel good. You are relaxed and you have a lot of energy stored up. You have retained the pleasurable experience of deep relaxation that you acquired in your fantasy. Whenever you are ready, slowly open your eyes. Take your time and enjoy this experience. Keep it with you throughout the day.

DAY 2

Make a contract with yourself. Resolve to make certain changes in your behavior. Decide what specific changes you want to make, then write down the steps you are going to take to accomplish your goal. For example, if you want to slow down when you drive, resolve to stay within the speed limit and to leave earlier for your destination. If you want to stop bringing work home, resolve to go in earlier or leave work later instead. Or if you wish to eat more slowly, take a definite lunch period and relax during lunch.

Look through the list in your Stress Notebook and select any items you would like to change by contracting with yourself to do so. Actually write up a brief contract in your notebook and record the times you breach your contract.

Review your Daily Stress Experiences sheet. Are you satisfied with the action you took in each instance? Do you think you could do better with what you learned today?

Learn to do the following general muscle relaxation procedure and do it for ten minutes each day. Note that it takes much practice and patience to acquire relaxation of the deep muscles. Avoid excessive tightening and overindulgence of the muscles in the neck and back areas to prevent spinal or muscle injuries or muscle spasms. Do the same for other muscle groups.

General Muscle Relaxation Procedure

1. Sit in a chair in a relaxed position.
2. Tense the feet by bending them toward the head as tightly as you can, causing the shins to feel very tight. Hold for a few seconds, then immediately relax.
3. Bend the feet by curling the toes away from the head as tightly as you can for a few seconds and immediately relax them. Repeat this with the legs fully extended.
4. Tighten your buttocks, hold for a few seconds, relax suddenly. Repeat three times.
5. Tighten your fists with your forearms facing upward and bend your wrists upward as tightly as you can and hold for a few seconds. Relax. Repeat this with the wrists bent downward. Sustain a few seconds and relax.
6. Curl the fingers of both hands and grasp the fingers of both hands like a hook. Pull as hard as you can, sustaining this action. Relax suddenly. Now open the left hand fully and make a fist with the right. Push the fist against the palm as hard as you can. Sustain for a few seconds, then relax suddenly. Change hands and repeat.
7. Bend your head forward so that your chin presses against your chest. Relax. Now bend the neck back as far as possible, then roll the neck to the right, then to the left. Now make a complete circular turn.
8. Raise your shoulders as high as possible, sustain for a few seconds, then drop them. Throw back the shoulders and relax.

9. Relax, then completely fill your lungs with air. Hold the air in your lungs for a couple of seconds, then breathe out slowly until you can't breathe anymore. Hold for a couple of seconds. Repeat this a few times.
10. Push your jaw forward forcefully and hold. Then relax quickly. Tighten your jaws, hold a few seconds, then relax. Wrinkle the forehead, hold, then relax. Blow up the cheeks, hold, then relax.
11. Protrude the tongue forcefully out of the mouth, then draw it back into the mouth, pressing against the roof of the mouth. Relax.
12. Tighten your stomach and hold it for a few seconds. Relax quickly. Place your hands, clasped, on your stomach and breathe in so as to inflate your stomach against the resistance of your hands. Relax.

Continue to practice your exercise plan every day.

DAY 3

1. Try noticing the following symptoms to tell when you are under stress:

   - rapid knee shaking
   - table tapping
   - feeling tight across your head
   - gritting or grinding your teeth
   - feeling a lump in your throat
   - muscle tightness

   At the first sign of these symptoms, either take a fast walk or try the meditation method on page 120 or the general muscle relaxation procedure on page 122.
2. If you have any of the symptoms in the list or others that you note by introspection, write them in your Stress Notebook and relate your course of action. Form the habit of reviewing each day's results and going back over previous days to compare your course of action.
3. Practice the meditation method for 20 minutes at the usual time and place every day. It is important that this be done at the same time each day, preferably when you are least apt to be disturbed and when it is quiet. This procedure is very relaxing and is an excellent way to combat insomnia resulting from stress.
4. Practice the general muscle relaxation procedure for 10 minutes each day. You will note that it can be done more quickly each day.
5. Continue doing your aerobic exercises every day.

DAY 4

1. Practice *hostility reduction* for 15 minutes today. Hostility is one of the most important and by far the most difficult of all the behavioral patterns to modify. Will Rogers once said, "People who fly into a rage always make a bad landing." Resolve today to modifying this pattern by practicing some of the tips given.

   If you are in bumper-to-bumper traffic, accept your fate. Use the standing breathing exercise on page 93 and the rapid muscle relaxation procedure, which you will learn on day 5, if you feel all keyed up.

   Don't make comments to belittle the ticket agent or bank teller when standing in line, because it is your heart and blood vessels that are being affected.

   Practice standing in a long movie or bank line and try starting up a conversation with someone. Use this opportunity to practice a short muscle relaxation procedure or breathing exercise.

   Carry a magazine, puzzle, book or short work items with you whenever you have to wait, such as at the doctor's office, movies, etc.

   When another motorist passes you or makes a dirty remark or sign, learn to ignore it and smile instead. Why let him be victorious in disturbing you? If you don't get upset, you are the winner. Instead, follow the advice of Thomas Jefferson, who said, "When angry, count ten before you speak; if very angry, a hundred."

2. Review your Stress Notebook and analyze the actions you have taken with each stress experience. Are you improving? Have you applied the muscle relaxation methods or breathing exercises to any of them?

3. Don't forget to practice the meditation and general muscle relaxation exercises each day. Are you sleeping more restfully? Are these techniques effective in relaxing you and relieving your stress? Remember, these procedures are like vintage wines—they get better with age.

4. Continue with your aerobic exercise program every day.

5. For 5 minutes each day practice the standing breathing exercise that is used in the 14-Day Quit-Smoking Plan (chapter 4). This is an upright method that has an advantage over the supine breathing exercise given in the same chapter in that it can be used throughout the day while standing.

6. If you have difficulty licking the traffic jam every day without demonstrating marked hostility, try taking a bus or train instead.

7. When a telephone caller make you angry, grasp the phone as tightly

as you can, count to 10 and release it suddenly. This is an excellent procedure that really works. Also practice this technique whenever a phone call creates tension.

DAY 5

Imitation is the copying of beneficial behavior patterns of other people who are faced with similar problems. This behavioral modification technique is quite effective and has its own niche in stress control therapy. Here are some hints for learning to use this method today:

1. Select certain people you suspect as being type B and use the same approach they do in handling various situations. For example, when one type B person was unduly taken to task for the way in which he handled an account, he very meekly answered the boss, "Thanks for calling this to my attention and for your comments. I will do as you suggested in the future." This made the boss feel important, and the employee totally avoided any cardiovascular trauma.
2. Don't hesitate in asking one of these type B people for advice regarding a particular problem.
3. Whenever you use this method, write it in your Stress Notebook and then indicate the results of this action.

More Tips to Reduce Stress

1. When you know that you will soon encounter a stressful event, evaluate the situation fully and practice it beforehand. In this way you can approach a stressful event with familiarity and confidence, thus diminishing the stressful effects.
2. After a stressful ordeal has passed, always rehabilitate yourself by using the general muscle relaxation procedure, the standing breathing exercise and the meditation method. Write the results in your Stress Notebook so you can refer to it.
3. Don't forget to practice the meditation method, general muscle relaxation procedure and standing breathing exercise today and every day without fail.
4. Practice the following rapid muscle relaxation procedure several times each day until you can perform it almost automatically. This is a short procedure that can be done in less than 30 seconds and is well adapted for immediate use during the day and whenever needed in stressful situations. It may also be useful in the 14-Day Heart-Saving Stop-Smoking Plan.

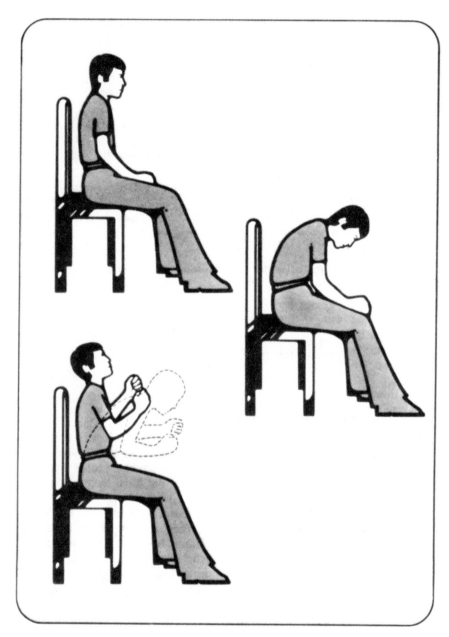

Rapid muscle relaxation procedure (30-second exercise).
    a. Sit straight up in a chair as shown in the following diagram, with the knees about 12 inches apart and legs slanting forward at an angle greater than 90 degrees.
    b. Unbutton your belt slightly to relieve the tension, loosen your tie and if you wear glasses or a watch, remove them.

   c. Sit straight and tall. Then suddenly collapse your body like a rag doll, your head forward and your spine rounded. Your hands will be on your knees.

   d. Concentrate on your right arm from your armpit to your fingertips for about 20 seconds, saying to yourself over and over again, "My right arm is heavy." Repeat with the left arm.

   e. Make a fist, then flex your arms. Now take a deep breath and open your eyes.

   f. In the same manner concentrate on making each leg heavy, then proceed to other parts of the body.

5. Practice the standing breathing exercise twice a day.
6. Did you exercise today? Remember, it must be done every day without fail.
7. Again review your Stress Notebook. How did you do today?

DAY 6

To reduce stress, it is important to develop different attitudes in stressful situations that you can't change. One way to do this is by using *buffers* against these situations. For instance, if you hate your job but are taking evening courses to learn computer programming, this will give you something to look forward to each time you encounter an unpleasant experience. The buffer in this instance might be thinking, "Well, at least this is only temporary until I complete my training," each time an unpleasant experience occurs.

Another way of using buffers is to substitute thoughts of unpleasant experiences of the day with thoughts of pleasant experiences. A reprimand by the boss may be buffered by a report from your doctor indicating that you are in excellent health. Try to think of other buffers you can use to reduce stress.

Make a poster with the words SLOW DOWN in large letters. Post this where you can see it during the workday. Each time you see it, do a standing breathing exercise.

Did you relax before eating when you came home from work today? If yes, good! If no, you'd better start right away.

Bring any work home with you? If no, super! If yes, you're making a big mistake.

Remember to do your meditation and your general relaxation procedures today. You will never regret learning these procedures, as they will reap great rewards. When you can do them almost automatically, you will possess a great weapon against stress.

Do a standing breathing exercise two or three times today. This exercise is also worth its weight in gold. Soon you will be able to do it at a moment's notice whenever stress is a problem.

Do the rapid muscle relaxation procedure a few times today. It only takes about 30 seconds.

DAY 7

Persistent unrelenting worry and fears of all kinds can produce a great deal of stress. They may involve such things as:

- Worry about whether you did a particular job right.
- Worry about your health. Every little sensation or ache may be interpreted as being something serious.
- Worry about getting old.
- Phobias of all kinds.
- Frightening recurring thoughts.
- Worry about germs.
- Worry about having an accident when driving.
- Fear of remaining unmarried.
- Worry about going out of town.
- Fears of being held up or mugged.

Thought-stopping is a very effective technique for overcoming these worries and fears. Here's how you do it.

Make a list in your Stress Notebook of any thoughts that are gnawing at you.

Purchase a calculator or watch alarm or the kind of pocket buzzer used to determine when a coin is due in a parking meter. Set this for about three minutes.

Meditate on the annoying thought and include the circumstances that precipitate it and everything you know about it. When the alarm or buzzer goes off, jump up suddenly or slap your face and yell *no* or *stop*.

Practice this for several days, then try it without an alarm or buzzer. Instead, interrupt the thought at will by yelling the word *no* or *stop* and slapping your face or wrist. Another novel idea is to place a rubber band around a finger (not too tight, please) and snap it when you yell the word *stop*.

How did you do at lunch today? Did you take a lunch break? If yes, good! If no, why not? Everyone is entitled to a lunch break. You must relax. Contract with yourself to take a lunch break. Record it in your Stress Notebook.

How long did your lunch break last? You must take at least forty-five minutes to an hour.

Did you eat slowly? If yes, you are learning, if no, why not? You must concentrate on eating slowly. Contract with yourself that you will chew each bite fifteen times, and record this in your Stress Notebook.

Do your usual meditation and general muscle relaxation procedures. Do a few standing breathing exercises today, also. Is your aerobic exercise program progressing according to plan?

Do the rapid muscle relaxation procedure a few times today. Is it getting easier and faster to perform? You can do the procedure four times in about two minutes.

In your Stress Notebook, review today's notations and collate them with the entire week. Do you note an improvement in coping with your stressful experiences? Review all your self-contracts. Do you have any breaches?

DAY 8

Poor management of time can be a major factor in the development of continual stress. You must put your house in order. Poor management of time leads to:

- missing deadlines
- chronic anxiety
- work backlogs
- lack of efficiency
- poor quality
- rushing
- reduction of quantity
- fatigue
- decreased morale
- constant work pressures

Resolve today to learn to manage time and not let time manage you by following these simple steps.

- Schedule your work more practically.
- Make priority lists. Rearrange the work from most important at the top to least important at the bottom, and begin at the top.
- Delegate. Start out by assigning the less important tasks, observing the finished product and progressively increasing the degree of responsibility.
- Make proper decisions. Evaluate the problems as they come along. If in doubt, ask the opinion of experienced employees or supervisors,

discuss problems at staff meetings, check previous decisions as to outcome and defer decisions if you are tired.

Make a list of all your activities for three days. Begin with rising in the morning and end at bedtime. Include what time the alarm went off; how long it took you to get out of bed, to shower and shave, to eat and get out of the house, to get to work; time spent on phone calls each day; time spent socializing; time spent at meetings; actual work time; time spent daydreaming; non-work-related time; time for coffee breaks and other activities, time watching television or listening to the radio and so on.

Analyze each item and allot time limits for activities such as phone conversations, getting ready for bed, getting ready to leave the house, lunch, coffee breaks and the like.

Set up a daily schedule for the meditation method, the general muscle relaxation procedure and the aerobic exercise plan similar to the following one. Incorporate this schedule into your daily itinerary for life. This will herein be referred to as the Daily Relaxation-Exercise Schedule.

Procedure	Mon	Tues	Wed	Thur	Fri	Sat	Sun
meditation	8 P.M.	8 P.M.	8 P.M.	8 P.M.	8 P.M.	8 P.M.	8 P.M.
muscle relaxation	4 P.M.	3 P.M.	3 P.M.	4 P.M.	4 P.M.	4 P.M.	3 P.M.
exercise program	7 A.M.	7 A.M.	7 A.M.	7 A.M.	7 A.M.	7 A.M.	7 A.M.

Practice the supine breathing exercise each day for five days. This exercise is performed in a lying-down position and takes much longer to perform than the standing breathing exercise. Although it would be awkward to perform during the day while pursuing your daily duties, the supine breathing exercise should be added to your armory for fighting stress, since it is very effective in counteracting anxiety and depression.

DAYS 9–14

1. Follow the Daily Relaxation-Exercise Schedule you prepared on Day 8.

   The general muscle relaxation procedure should be done for ten to fifteen minutes each day. This method should also be used whenever you have a day of increased stress with accompanying muscle tension, fatigue, headache, fears and intestinal upsets. It is useful as a routine for anyone with high blood pressure (see chapter 5) and should be used to treat insomnia. Excessive tightening and overindulgence of the muscles in the neck and back areas must be avoided to prevent spinal or muscle injuries or muscle spasms.

Perform the meditation method for twenty minutes every day— permanently. This should become a way of life. Remember, this procedure must be done in a quiet room at the same time each day. Meditation places you in a state of deep relaxation and puts you in control. In this way the fight-or-flight reaction is curtailed. This method is also excellent for blood pressure reduction (see chapter 5) and is very helpful in reducing the stresses associated with smoking.

Exercise regularly for at least fifteen to twenty minutes each day without fail.

2. Perform the standing breathing exercise twice a day. By now this method should be well learned. This exercise should be used to counteract or reduce anxiety and depression throughout the day. It is also useful in coping with the stresses and cravings for a cigarette during the 14-Day Heart-Saving Quit-Smoking program.

3. Perform the supine breathing exercise once a day.

4. Perform the rapid muscle relaxation procedure for a few minutes each day, so that it can be done on a moment's notice whenever you become involved in a stressful experience. Record it in your Stress Notebook when you use it to cope with a stressful event.

5. Participate in the 14-Day Heart-Saving Exercise program.

6. Continue making entries in your Stress Notebook, analyzing them daily to follow your progress. A careful review will tell you which methods work best for you. In this manner you can eliminate some of the methods and practice the effective ones until they become second nature. Also continue contracting with yourself until you effectively modify some of your undesirable behavior patterns.

7. Repeat your study of the material on behavioral modification given each day in item #1. This is best done by restudying one topic each day. Using the notes from your Stress Notebook, determine if they have been helpful. In addition, check to see where they might have been useful if you had thought to use them.

8. Are you scrutinizing your activities? Are you still bringing work home? If you are, try to determine why. Is it because your job really depends on it? Are you nurturing your deadline habit? Is it due to poor time management? By this process, you can identify the root of the problem and determine the best solution.

Are you taking a proper lunch break yet or are you procrastinating? Again, can you trace the source? Can it be poor time management, trying to get as many things into a day as you possibly can, or is it your deadline pattern? You must convince yourself that this break is important because it gives you time to relax, it breaks your work cycle and it changes your life pattern. If you are taking a lunch break, are you eating slowly? Now is the time to try the suggestion of chewing each bite about fifteen times.

Have you begun to relax for an hour when you first come home prior to eating a big meal, or are you procrastinating again? You must break the cycle now!

Have you begun to slow down while driving? while walking? Ask yourself, "Where am I going in such a hurry?" Did you put up the sign with the big letters SLOW DOWN where you can see it each day? If you haven't done it yet, contract to slow down and put it in your notebook.

How is your hostility pattern doing? Are you biting your tongue when someone makes a remark to you and using one of the relaxation techniques? Are you carrying a magazine, puzzle, book, newspaper or some work with you when you have to wait in line or in a reception room?

Are you using the technique of thought-stopping to overcome your worries and phobic thoughts? During this week practice this several times a day.

More tips to reduce stress.

When you know you will soon encounter a stressful event, evaluate the situation fully and practice it beforehand. In this way you can approach a stressful event with familiarity and confidence, thus diminishing the stressful effects.

If you are going to the hospital for a major or minor procedure, inquire of the doctor, nurse or a friend who previously had the procedure as to what to expect. It is the fear of the unknown that leads to severe stress. When a doctor makes you sign that frightening consent form that enumerates all the evils that may befall you, *don't panic*. Merely ask the frequency with which the doctor has actually seen these complications. You will be surprised to find how rare they are. These all-inclusive forms are a result of the malpractice age, with attempts to cover all bases.

Join an active part-time organization such as a voluntary fire organization, voluntary ambulance corps, charitable organization or church group.

Develop a home project, such as a part-time business venture, building a den, writing a book, working on a school project with your children and so on.

YOUR STRESS-CONTROL PRESCRIPTION FOR A HEALTHY HEART

The control of stress is a lifelong project that requires constant surveillance and continual perseverance. The 14-Day Heart-Saving Stress Control Plan provides you with the necessary weaponry to enable you to recognize the symptoms of stress, to identify events that precipitate stress and to apply appropriate stress-reducing techniques and preventive measures.

Chapter Seven

Vitamins, Minerals,

Trace Elements

and Your Heart

> *. . . One ought to be acquainted with the powers of juices, and what action each of them has upon man. . . .*
>
> —Hippocrates

In recent years tremendous progress has been made in understanding the role that vitamins and minerals play in preventing cardiovascular disease. Many new studies indicate that spcific vitamins and minerals may be important in cardiovascular health.

VITAMINS AND CARDIOVASCULAR DISEASE

Vitamin A

Restricting your dairy products with the 14-Day Heart-Saving Menu Plan may significantly reduce your total intake of vitamin A. Therefore, it is important that you eat adequate amounts of vitamin-A-rich foods and take a supplement if your intake of vitamin-rich foods is inadequate. The recommended daily allowance (RDA) of vitamin A for adult males is 1000 retinol equivalents (5000 IUs) and 800 retinol equivalents (4000 IUs) for females.* Serious toxicity may occur in adults with intakes of vitamin A in

---

*Recently the expression of the vitamin A values in foods as International Units (IUs) was changed to the equivalent weight of retinol, with 1 retinol equaling 3.33 IUs.

excess of 15,000 retinol equivalents (50,000 IUs). It is with this danger in mind that the Committee on Dietary Allowances of the National Research Council indicates that a daily ingestion of more than 7500 retinol equivalents (25,000 IUs) is not prudent.

The following foods are high in vitamin A. Even modest amounts of some of these vegetables will easily satisfy the RDA requirements.

- apricots
- broccoli
- spinach
- carrots
- butternut squash
- sweet potato
- parsley
- cress, garden
- pumpkin
- kale

Other foods with significant amounts of vitamin A include leaf lettuce, mustard greens, corn, green beans, peas, watermelon, beet greens, tomatoes with skins and muskmelons.

Consider taking vitamin A supplements on days that you do not eat enough vitamin-A-rich foods. Since vitamin A is one of the fat-soluble vitamins, it is important that some fat be present in your diet at the same time that you are ingesting vitamin-A-rich foods or vitamin A supplements; otherwise the vitamin may not be absorbed from the intestine. Do not, however, ingest more than the recommended amounts indicated on page 134.

Vitamin B$_6$

This vitamin may play a prominent role in cardiovascular health. It has been reported to lower cholesterol and triglyceride levels, improve glucose tolerance and inhibit the development of atherosclerotic plaques in the arteries of laboratory animals on atherosclerosis-producing diets. When monkeys were made deficient in this vitamin, they developed atherosclerosis. The need for this vitamin is greatly increased when protein in the diet is increased. The RDA is about 2.2 milligrams of vitamin B$_6$ for women and 2.0 milligrams for men. Much larger amounts, however, were used in the scientific studies described.

Until recently it was believed that none of the water-soluble vitamins was toxic, because they were quickly removed from the body. Then in

1983 seven cases of vitamin B₆ toxicity involving the nervous system were described in the *New England Journal of Medicine* in persons consuming from 1000 to 3000 times the RDA for from two to forty months. Another report followed in the same journal in 1984, of a thirty-four-year-old woman who developed toxicity from taking only 500 milligrams daily for a prolonged period of time. Amounts above 200 milligrams each day are best avoided, since there is a paucity of well-designed studies for intakes between this amount and 1000 milligrams. Foods containing significant amounts of vitamin B₆ include the following:

mackerel
halibut
tuna
salmon
wheat germ
soybeans
sunflower seed kernels
chicken, light meat
buckwheat flour
brewer's yeast
brown rice
banana
peanuts
whole grains

Vitamin C (Ascorbic Acid)

Vitamin C may play an important role in cardiovascular health. It increases the "good" cholesterol, decreases the total cholesterol in the blood and increases the activity of certain substances in the blood that dissolve clots within blood vessels. In a 1981 study men with coronary artery disease treated with vitamin C for six weeks showed an increase in "good" cholesterol and a decrease in the total cholesterol and "bad" cholesterol in the blood. A Hungarian study in 1977 reported a 10 to 15 percent reduction in cholesterol in twenty healthy males who were fed vitamin C. In animals fewer atherosclerotic plaques form in the arteries when vitamin C is added to the diet. Moreover, certain products that are present in the blood called *free radicals* can cause damage to the artery walls. These arise as a result of oxidation of various substances, such as polyunsaturated fatty acids and from the effects of radiation. Fortunately, antioxidant substances such as vitamin C, vitamin E and selenium can destroy these free radicals.

The RDA for vitamin C is given as 60 milligrams each day, but this level is far too low to increase the "good" cholesterol and lower the total cholesterol and triglycerides in the blood or to counteract the effect of the free radical concentration, since amounts in excess of 500 milligram have been used in most of the scientific studies to effect such a change. Although there have been some reports of adverse effects with megadoses, such as physical dependency, excessive iron absorption, high uric acid levels in the urine and impaired activity of the bacteria-fighting white blood corpuscles, the number of reported cases in comparison to the number taking the vitamin appears quite small.

Before taking megadoses of this or any vitamin, you should consult your physician. Anyone on large doses of vitamin C should have a blood test for iron and a urine test for uric acid.

Vitamin C is quite unstable and may be destroyed or lost by cooking and storage, and cigarette smoking has been reported to lower vitamin C levels. Foods with significant amounts of vitamin C include the following:

orange juice
orange, peeled
grapefruit juice
grapefruit, sections
lemon
lime
papaya
tangerine juice
tomato juice
acerola juice
muskmelon
broccoli
strawberries
watercress, chopped
green peppers
potato, boiled
spinach, leaf
Brussels sprouts
cabbage
turnip greens

Vitamin E

Independent studies conducted in 1979, 1982 and 1983 revealed an increase in the level of the "good" cholesterol in the blood of people who consumed substantial amounts of vitamin E. A study published in the

Journal of Clinical Investigation in 1976 reported a reduction in the clumping of platelets, the tiny cellular structures in the blood that promote clotting. This could prevent small clots from forming in the arteries that may give rise to heart attack, stroke or other related disease. The requirements for vitamin E increase when a person eats more polyunsaturated fats, but the foods that are high in polyunsaturates, such as vegetable oils, margarines and shortening, are also the richest source of this vitamin. Vitamin E also appears to operate in concert with vitamin C and selenium as antioxidants against the free radicals, which may damage blood vessels.

Vitamin E has been reported to be relatively nontoxic as compared to the other fat-soluble vitamins, A and D. Although there have been inconsistent reports of adverse reactions occurring with intakes of 400 to 1000 IUs, most adults appear to tolerate these doses without any problem. Anyone planning to take large doses of vitamin E should check with a physician. The following foods are good sources of vitamin E:

> wheat germ oil
> vegetable oils: safflower, corn, soy, peanut, cottonseed, sunflower, etc.
> nuts: pecans, almonds, walnuts, pistachios, hazelnuts, peanuts
> seeds: sunflower seed kernels, pumpkin seeds

MINERALS, TRACE ELEMENTS AND CARDIOVASCULAR DISEASE

Minerals

The hardness of drinking water appears to be due to its calcium and magnesium content. The more of these minerals present, the harder the water. This relationship assumed prominence when an association between the hardness of drinking water and cardiovascular disease was reported: it was alleged that an increased incidence of cardiovascular disease was present in those areas where the water was deficient in these minerals (soft-water areas) and a decreased incidence was present where the mineral content was increased (hard-water areas). These findings were refuted by other studies that failed to show such a correlation. Now, however, a quantitative reevaluation indicates that there appears to be a strong correlation between the amount of magnesium in the water and the incidence of cardiovascular disease.

Although a relationship between magnesium and cardiovascular disease has not been definitely proved, there is strong supportive evidence for such a link. A 1962 study revealed 855 cardiac deaths per 100,000 men in Glasgow, Scotland, where the drinking water is soft, as compared to 581 deaths per 100,000 in London, where the water is hard. In 1966 a similar study showed 300 cardiac deaths per 100,000 men in Lincoln, Nebraska, where the water is hard, as compared to 800 per 100,000 in Savannah, Georgia, where the water is soft. Another report in 1976 indicated that magnesium deficiency may increase the risk of death after a heart attack in soft-water areas. A French autopsy study showed a markedly lower magnesium content in hearts of heart-attack victims as compared to those dying from other causes. Dogs made deficient in magnesium can develop cardiac arrest. Another study in 1981 with magnesium-deficient rats revealed an increase in total cholesterol, "bad" cholesterol and triglycerides and a decrease in "good" cholesterol. There is also some evidence that magnesium may combine with some fats in the small intestine so they cannot be digested.

Causes of magnesium deficiency other than dietary consumption include alcoholism, kidney disease, severe and prolonged diarrhea, defects in absorption of food, endocrine disturbances and uncontrolled diabetes. The RDA for magnesium is currently 300 milligrams a day for females and 350 for males. Scientists at Downstate Medical Center of the State University of New York indicate that this amount might be okay if our intake of calcium, phosphates and vitamin D were not so high. Otherwise as much as 500 to 600 milligrams per day may be required. The toxic effects from ingesting large amounts of magnesium occur primarily in people with serious kidney disease and in association with a disease of pregnancy called eclampsia. The ninth edition of the *Recommended Daily Allowances* manual indicates that there is no evidence that large oral intakes of magnesium are harmful if a person's kidney function is normal, but that amounts in the 3000- to 5000-milligram range have a laxative effect. *AMA Drug Evaluations* indicate that magnesium sulfate may be toxic in amounts over 10,000 milligrams, particularly with prolonged use. *Remember, if you have a kidney disease, check with your physician before taking magnesium supplements.* Fats and refined sugars make a very small contribution to the magnesium intake, as they are almost devoid of magnesium. The common foods from most to least that contain magnesium are as follows:

nuts
cereals
seafoods
meats
legumes
vegetables
dairy products
refined sugars

Trace Elements

The trace elements of importance in cardiovascular disease include *chromium* and *selenium.*

CHROMIUM

This metal plays an essential role in sugar metabolism because it forms an integral part of the glucose tolerance factor (GTF), a chemical complex that combines with insulin, permitting it to work properly. The beneficial effects of chromium in cardiovascular disease and diabetes have been demonstrated in many excellent studies. It raises the "good" cholesterol, lowers the "bad" cholesterol, lowers total cholesterol, improves the action of insulin and inhibits atherosclerotic plaques.

In a study published in 1981 at West Virginia University School of Medicine, twenty-three healthy men given chromium over a twelve-week period showed a significant increase in their "good" cholesterol levels, with a trend toward lower triglyceride levels. A 1982 experimental study on rabbits fed high-cholesterol diets and also given chromium showed a 50 percent reduction in atherosclerotic plaques, and another study also using rabbits showed a regression of cholesterol-induced plaques. A ten-year study published in 1977 revealed a higher mortality from coronary artery disease in the eastern area of the country than in the western area, where chromium in the drinking water was higher.

Chromium deficiency probably occurs in humans, since various studies have shown an improvement in a person's glucose tolerance following chromium supplementation. The refining of various foods such as sugar and flour may significantly reduce their chromium content. If you eat a diet high in refined sugar, your chromium will be rapidly used up. Moreover, high-carbohydrate diets in general will enhance chromium excretion in the urine.

The tentative RDA for chromium in adults is 50 to 200 micrograms. Trivalent chromium has a low order of toxicity with a wide margin of safety, and various studies have shown that taking 150 to 200 micrograms of chromium is completely safe and very effective. Impaired glucose tolerance was improved in diabetics not dependent on insulin and in older people on daily supplements of 150 micrograms of inorganic chromium.

Brewer's yeast and certain spices have the highest concentrations of chromium. Significant amounts are also found in certain meats, fish, mushrooms, shellfish, skim milk, cheeses and whole grains. Liver and kidney are relatively high in chromium but have a high cholesterol content. Chromium also leaches out from foods cooked in stainless-steel cookware.

Good results have been reported with GTF supplements, also known as glucose tolerance factor chromium. Brewer's yeast tablets may also be used to supplement the diet.

SELENIUM

Selenium's role in cardiovascular health derives from its function as part of the enzyme glutathione peroxidase, which is present in red blood corpuscles to protect the cells against damage by certain products of oxidation called *free radical* or *superoxides*. These free radicals can damage artery walls. Selenium performs this antioxidant function in concert with vitamin C and vitamin E.

The RDA for selenium that is safe for adults is from 50 to 200 micrograms daily. It is recommended that you not exceed this level, because selenium is very toxic. The content of selenium in food is related to the food's protein content and geographical origin. Therefore, foods low in protein would be almost devoid of it. In areas where the selenium content is low, the fruits, vegetables and animal products are low in selenium, and vice versa. This is the reason it is difficult to ascribe selenium values to foods in general. Municipal water supplies are very low in selenium, regardless of the water source.

In general, loss from cooking is small. Good sources of selenium include brewer's yeast, seafoods and meats, while wheat germ and other grains are more variable in content. Liver and kidney are good sources but cannot be used because of their high cholesterol content, and fruits and vegetables in general contain very little of this metal.

TIPS

1. Check with your physician before taking large doses of vitamins or minerals above the recommended levels. Your doctor is in a good position to evaluate whether the dose you are contemplating taking would be detrimental to your present physical condition. Moreover, patients taking medications should check with their physician before taking vitamin or mineral supplements as there are complex interactions between various drugs and nutrients.
2. Always take fat-soluble vitamins A, D, E and K with meals containing some fat. These vitamins must dissolve in fat to be properly absorbed in the intestinal tract. For example, if you take any of these vitamins with a bowl of fruit and a glass of skim milk, very little of the

vitamins will be absorbed. Take them with any meal containing fat, whether it be an oil-and-vinegar-dressed salad at the evening meal or just toast with margarine at breakfast.

3. When taking zinc supplements or zinc-rich foods, avoid taking any chromium supplements like GTF, brewer's yeast, etc., at the same time. Chromium and zinc share a common absorption system in which an excess of one may interfere with absorption of the other.

4. When taking chromium, don't eat foods rich in iron, because they share a common carrier for transport in the body. Again, an excess of one could affect the transport of the other.

5. If you begin a high-fiber diet, eat additional amounts of foods containing zinc, magnesium, iron, phosphorus and calcium. There appears to be a decrease in absorption of these elements when eating a high-fiber diet.

6. When you eat vitamin-C-rich foods or supplements, take them at the same time you take your calcium-rich foods or supplements for maximum absorption of the latter. If you want to cut down on your calcium absorption, take the vitamin C at a different time or cut down on your calcium intake. Also take your iron supplements at the same time you eat your vitamin-C-rich foods or supplements if you are anemic. Vitamin C also provides for maximal absorption of iron. If, however, you are taking large doses of vitamin C and taking iron supplements, have frequent blood tests to avoid absorbing too much iron.

Chapter Eight

The 14-Day Heart-Saving

Diabetes Control Plan

*He that will not apply new remedies
must expect new evils. . . .*
—Francis Bacon

WHAT IS DIABETES?

When we eat sugars and starches, chemicals in our intestinal tract convert them to *glucose,* a type of sugar the body uses for fuel. After the glucose is absorbed into the circulation, the body may either burn it right away to supply energy or it may store it for later use. In order for the body to do either, a hormone produced by the pancreas, called *insulin,* must be present.

Diabetics, however, are unable to use the glucose properly, either because their bodies do not make enough insulin or because they are unable to use the insulin that is made. Therefore, large amounts of glucose accumulates in the blood (hyperglycemia), because the body is unable either to use it or store it. This forces the body to metabolize fats and proteins for energy in place of glucose and forces the kidneys to work overtime in order to spill the excess sugar into the urine.

Two major types of diabetes have recently been established by the National Diabetes Data Group. *Type I* is called *insulin-dependent diabetes* and *Type II* is known as *noninsulin-dependent diabetes.* Type I, the most severe, occurs in childhood and accounts for 10 percent of all cases of diabetes. Because people with this type produce almost no insulin, they need regular injections of this hormone to preserve life. The symptoms of Type I appear suddenly and include severe thirst, frequent urination, a craving for food, weight loss, weakness, behavioral changes and perhaps even coma.

By contrast, Type II diabetes more commonly occurs in middle age or later and accounts for most of the remaining 90 percent of cases. People with this type of diabetes produce insulin, but in much smaller or less effective quantities than normal. Patients are often helped by diet alone or with oral medication. They don't need injections unless it's necessary to control their high blood sugar levels.

About 80 percent of Type II diabetics are obese, and their symptoms come on more gradually than in Type I diabetics. They may suffer from increased thirst, frequent urination, increased appetite, tiredness, itching, leg cramps, sleepiness, skin and urinary tract infections. Many Type II patients, however, have no symptoms at all and are detected by routine screening tests. These patients may be helped by diet, insulin or oral diabetic drugs.

THE EFFECT OF DIABETES ON THE HEART

The leading cause of death in diabetics is cardiovascular disease. Diabetes was reported as one of the risk factors in coronary artery disease by the Framingham (1972), New Bedford (1965) and Tecumseh studies (1965). While this relationship between diabetes and coronary disease is clear in Western cultures, it is not so apparent in other peoples.

Atherosclerotic heart disease and heart attacks are five times more prevalent in diabetics. Autopsies on diabetics reveal a marked prevalence of atherosclerotic plaques in the coronary arteries, as compared to non-diabetics. The disease is more severe and shows up at an earlier age among diabetics, also. However, heart attacks are uncommon in non-diabetic females prior to the menopause, but they are nearly as common in diabetic females as they are in diabetic males. Strokes, kidney failure, gangrene of the lower extremities and blindness are also seen in diabetics much more frequently than in nondiabetics.

HIGH BLOOD PRESSURE AND DIABETES

High blood pressure occurs in adult diabetics far more frequently than in the general population. The longer a person is diabetic, the greater the chances of having high blood pressure. About 70 percent of people who have had the disease for over thirty-five years also have high blood pressure. Why this is true is not entirely clear, but the effect of diabetes on the blood vessels of the kidneys is certainly one of the reasons. Others are the greater incidence of obesity, accelerated atherosclerosis and kidney infections among diabetics. Oral contraceptives containing estrogen may cause both high blood pressure and diabetes, both of which improve after stopping use of the pill.

Many of the drugs used to treat high blood pressure have been shown to raise the blood sugar levels. For example, thiazide diuretics frequently raise the blood sugar level. Beta blockers may also raise it. Both drugs have also been implicated in lowering the "good" cholesterol and raising the triglyceride levels. The risk for a person having both diabetes and high blood pressure at the same time is significantly greater than the sum of the risk factors for each disease.

WEIGHT REDUCTION AND DIABETES

In the years prior to our present understanding of diabetes, obesity was recognized as a predisposing factor in Type II diabetes. Recent statistics indicate that obesity is present in about two-thirds of diabetics between the ages of thirty and sixty-five. Since weight loss alone may normalize both the blood sugar level and triglyceride level, weight reduction must be the major goal in the treatment of overweight diabetics.

Low-Fat, Low-Cholesterol Diet

Since diabetics have an unusually high prevalence of premature cardiovascular disease and frequently show disturbances in their blood triglyceride, cholesterol and "bad" cholesterol levels, doctors recommend a diet consisting of not more than 30 percent of the total calories from fat, not more than 10 percent from saturated fat and approximately 55 percent from complex carbohydrates. The 14-Day Heart-Saving Menu Plan given in chapter 3 satisfies these recommendations.

Exercise

Exercise improves the utilization of carbohydrates and fats in diabetes, and it has also been shown to increase the effectiveness of insulin. When you exercise, your body burns up sugar. People on insulin who exercise regularly find that their insulin requirements are decreased. Diabetics should avoid strenuous exercise, as it may cause the blood sugar to drop to an abnormally low level, called *hypoglycemia*, particularly diabetics on insulin therapy. Exercise is also very valuable in helping diabetics lose and maintain weight.

ADVERSE EFFECTS OF ORAL DIABETIC DRUGS

An eight-year multicenter study by the University Group Diabetes Program reported in 1970 and 1976 that administration of the two oral hypoglycemic drugs tested (tolbutamide and phenformin) resulted in significantly more deaths from cardiovascular disease than diet alone or insulin alone. The controversy following this study led to a reevaluation of the data by the Biometric Society, which essentially upheld the observations and conclusions. Most experts agree that no studies have demonstrated any beneficial effects of oral hypoglycemic drugs in preventing the long-term complications of diabetes and recommend that dietary means should be tried first, insulin added when necessary and oral hypoglycemic drugs considered for Type II individuals only when diet and weight reduction prove to be ineffective and the patient refuses insulin therapy. There is also a long list of other side effects associated with oral hypoglycemic agents that vary from jaundice and blood disorders to liver and gastrointestinal disorders.

Can Blood Sugar Be Lowered Without Drugs?

The recommended first-line medical treatment for all types of diabetes is diet modification, with weight reduction when obesity is present. Weight reduction alone or in some cases just caloric restriction frequently normalizes the blood sugar level.

High-fiber diets are also being used to treat diabetes. Scientists have noted for many years that diabetes is rare in societies that eat foods high in fiber, such as in some African tribes. African city dwellers whose diets are low in fiber have a much higher incidence of diabetes. In countries where the fiber content of the diet is low, such as the United States and England, there is a much greater incidence of diabetes. Many scientific studies published from 1974 to 1984 reported that substantial lowering of the blood sugar level and decreased need for insulin or oral hypoglycemic drugs can be achieved with an increase in dietary fiber in both Type I and Type II diabetes. Evidently insoluble fibers, such as guar (a gumlike substance extracted from the clusterbean) and pectin (a gelatinous substance present in the skins of fruits), delay the rise in blood sugar that usually occurs following a carbohydrate-rich meal. Today many diabetics may be able to eliminate their insulin or oral medications and control their blood sugar through the use of a high-fiber diet. Moreover, when the high-fiber diet is combined with a low-fat low-cholesterol diet, the blood cholesterol, triglycerides and sugar levels are all reduced.

Research on the role of chromium in diabetes control is also promising. This trace element, discussed fully in chapter 7, is important in glucose metabolism because it forms an integral part of the glucose tolerance factor (GTF), a chemical complex that combines with insulin, permitting the latter to work properly. Several scientific investigations showed a significant improvement in glucose tolerance in both Type II diabetics and in older people on daily chromium supplements. Chromium appears to have other benefits, such as raising the "good" cholesterol levels, decreasing the blood cholesterol and inhibiting atherosclerotic plaques.

THE 14-DAY HEART-SAVING DIABETES CONTROL PLAN

The 14-Day Heart-Saving Diabetes Control Plan contains all the basic principles to assist you and your physician in successfully lowering your blood sugar. These include:

1. reducing your weight to normal
2. eating a low-fat, low-cholesterol, low-sodium, calorie-restricted diet
3. adding fiber to the diet
4. supplementing the diet with chromium and other nutrients
5. exercising regularly
6. avoiding estrogen-containing oral contraceptives
7. avoiding thiazide diuretics, beta blockers and other drugs for treating high blood pressure whenever possible

A word of caution: If you are presently on a diabetic medication or diet, do not begin this program without getting your doctor's approval. Ask your doctor to read this program and then check your progress periodically. If you are on insulin, it is important that both you and your physician be aware that the high-fiber diet may dramatically decrease your insulin requirements and may require frequent blood sugar determinations at the beginning of the program. This also holds true for oral hypoglycemic agents.

DAY 1

If you are overweight, study the Low-Fat Low-Cholesterol Weight Reduction Plan today (see Appendix A). Schedule a program on your calendar to lose about two to three pounds each week. Be persistent and stick to the program, because weight reduction is critical to effectively lower both the blood sugar and triglyceride levels. Moreover, weight reduction alone may completely control both these factors. If you also have high blood pressure, then it is doubly important that you lose weight, since the presence of both risk factors constitutes a dangerous combination.

DAY 2

Study the 14-Day Heart-Saving Menu Plan today. Next, schedule this plan on your calendar so that you can learn how to lower the total cholesterol, "bad" cholesterol and triglyceride levels in your blood; raise the "good" cholesterol levels and begin to gradually change your dietary life-style.

Study chapter 7 on vitamins, minerals and trace elements so that you become aware of the amounts that are recommended for good cardiovascular and diabetic health.

DAY 3

Begin to incorporate the high-fiber diet into your daily menus. Start by reading about the principles of the high-fiber diet on pages 49–50 and study the ways to increase your fiber and starch intake on page 62. (Remember to check with your doctor as recommended.) This must be diligently learned but slowly incorporated into your diet. Your ultimate goal is an intake of 50 grams of fiber each day, but this is to be done gradually by starting out the first week with 30 grams and increasing 5 grams each week until you are consuming about 50 grams. Tables that list the amount of fiber in common foods are included in Appendix E. The reason for adding fiber gradually is to avoid the adverse effects of a sudden increase, which may include abdominal cramps, bloating and diarrhea.

DAY 4

Study the section on chromium on page 140. Learn all about chromium and its functions in the body and how to increase your dietary intake. Supplement your diet so that you get about 150 micrograms of chromium daily but no more if your doctor agrees.

DAY 5

Begin a regular exercise program today. Remember to take the Health Check Quiz in chapter 2 and, if necessary, get clearance from your doctor. Exercise lowers the blood sugar level and may decrease the amount of insulin required to lower the blood sugar. Select an aerobic exercise program from the 14-Day Heart-Saving Exercise Plan in chapter 2, incorporate a specific time in your schedule to exercise and exercise regularly without fail. Avoid strenuous exercise, as it may cause hypoglycemia, particularly in diabetics taking insulin. This is characterized by the sudden onset of clammy skin, pale coloration, irritability, confusion, nervousness and headache. Always carry a sugar food product like a bar of candy, sugar cubes or orange juice, and take some at the first sign of any of these symptoms.

DAY 6

Modify any other risk factors that you may have. Since premature cardiovascular disease is a common complication of diabetes and the leading cause of death, it is important to control all the associated risk factors.

If you are a smoker, try to stop cold turkey. If you are unsuccessful, study the 14-Day Heart-Saving Quit-Smoking Plan in chapter 4 and set a date on your calendar to begin the two-week program. It is extremely important to quit smoking, since it is one of the major risk factors; studies show that the "good" cholesterol will stay down if a person smokes even with regular exercise, modified diet and loss of weight.

If you have high blood pressure, study the 14-Day Heart-Saving Blood Pressure Control Plan in chapter 5 and schedule it on your calendar. Remember, don't just go off your blood pressure medication but check with your doctor.

DAY 7

Continue modifying any risk factors.

If you have a stressful occupation or a stressful home life, set a date on your calendar to begin the 14-Day Heart-Saving Stress Control Plan in chapter 6.

Under your doctor's direction, stop taking estrogen-containing contraceptives that raise the blood sugar level and elevate the blood pressure. Have him substitute other medications for thiazide diuretics, beta blockers and other blood pressure-lowering drugs that may raise the blood sugar level, increase the blood cholesterol and triglyceride levels and lower the "good" cholesterol level.

DAYS 8–14

1. Continue with your weight reduction program. This must be done almost religiously, because weight reduction alone may completely normalize your blood sugar and triglycerides and decrease or eliminate your need for insulin or oral agents.
2. Continue learning the principles of the 14-Day Heart-Saving Diet Plan in chapter 3 and the vitamin and mineral recommendations given in chapter 7.
3. Begin adding 35 grams of fiber to your diet this week, and continue adding an additional 5 grams each week until an intake of about 50 grams is reached.
4. Exercise regularly.
5. Put the stress reduction techniques from chapter 6 to work whenever a stressful event occurs.
6. Continue modifying any other risk factors you may have: smoking, high blood pressure, stress, etc.

YOUR PRESCRIPTION FOR A LOWER BLOOD SUGAR LEVEL

If you follow these recommendations, in most instances you will either normalize your blood sugar and triglyceride levels without the need for insulin or oral hypoglycemic agents or be able to maintain yourself at a significantly lower dose of the drugs. So get started immediately.

Chapter Nine

Answers to Your

Questions About

the 14-Day

Heart-Saving Program

Knowledge . . . is the great sun in the firmament.
Life and power are scattered with all its beams.
—Daniel Webster

What is *angina pectoris?*

This is a term derived from the Latin meaning "pain in the chest." It refers to tightness, pressure or a feeling of suffocation usually in the center of the chest, frequently accompanied by a spread of this discomfort to the neck, jaw, shoulder, arm or hand. It is caused by an insufficient amount of oxygen getting to the heart muscle because of severely narrowed coronary arteries. When the oxygen and nutrient needs of the heart increase, as with physical exertion, anxiety, heavy meals, cold weather and the like, the narrowed coronary circulation is unable to keep up with the demand, and anginal pain occurs.

Is atherosclerosis a reversible process?

Yes! According to both experimental and indirect clinical evidence. Many scientists have demonstrated a progressive removal of fats from atherosclerotic plaques that had been induced experimentally in laboratory animals. Autopsy studies on prisoners dying in concentration camps where the total caloric intake is significantly below normal revealed far less atherosclerosis in the arteries than in people of the same age and sex who were never in concentration camps. The same relationship was also found in people with chronic wasting diseases. Finally, yellow skin deposits called *xanthomas* that bear a close similarity to atherosclerotic plaques may disappear when the blood cholesterol level is significantly reduced.

What are the warning signs of a heart attack?

These are the most common warning signs. If one or more are present, get to the nearest hospital emergency room, preferably by ambulance. Commit these signs to memory, because they may save your life. Don't delay by attributing the pain to indigestion or muscle pain. There is too much at stake to take the risk. Don't gamble with your life.

1. heavy, uncomfortable pressure or squeezing pain in the middle of the chest (behind the breastbone) of a prolonged nature
2. spreading or radiating pain to the arm, shoulder, neck, jaw or teeth
3. severe pain in the chest, pit of the stomach or shoulders
4. cold sweats, with or without pressure or pain
5. shortness of breath, with or without chest discomfort
6. nausea and/or vomiting

Must I give up my predinner drink?

Absolutely not! A drink a day may actually keep a heart attack away, according to recent studies; the Honolulu Heart Study of 7,705 Japanese men living in Hawaii reported twice as many heart attacks in teetotalers than in men who had one or two drinks per day. This effect appears to derive from the ability of alcohol to raise the good cholesterol. This association was confirmed by several independent studies that included either American men, Swedish men, Italian men or marathon runners.

Another way alcohol may prevent heart disease comes from its ability to prevent blood clots from forming within the walls of the coronary arteries. According to researchers from the Royal Free Hospital in London, small amounts of alcohol stop the tiny cells called platelets from sticking together to form clots.

Before taking any alcohol with your evening meal, first check with your doctor. Alcohol may seriously aggravate many medical conditions, such as alcoholism, gout, liver disease, diabetes and gastrointestinal disease, and can interact with many medications.

If one or two drinks have this effect, wouldn't several drinks even further reduce the number of heart attacks?

Sorry, but when alcohol is imbibed in large quantities, it may cause sudden death or have other devastating effects. A study conducted in Chicago in 1977 suggested that sudden death was increased in an industrial group that had more than five drinks per day. The mechanism of sudden death appears to be triggered by severe rhythm disturbances of the heart caused by the increased alcohol consumption.

Doesn't alcohol raise the triglyceride level?

Yes and no. In most instances one or two drinks will not raise the triglyceride level provided a person is not overweight, but this is not so for all people. If a person is overweight, it is necessary to reduce the weight to normal prior to using alcohol. Remember, two drinks also contribute about 280 calories. Have your blood tested for triglycerides prior to drinking and several days after drinking to determine if the alcohol has any significant effect on your triglyceride level. If it does, then don't drink.

Several articles in the press link coffee drinking to an increased incidence of heart attacks. Should I stop drinking coffee?

The answer is no, according to a 1974 publication by Drs. Dawber, Kannel and Gordon of the famous Framingham study. They evaluated 1,992 men and 2,500 women over a twelve-year period and showed that coffee drinking is not a factor in the development of atherosclerotic heart disease. A recent Norwegian study in 1983, however, presents evidence that the more coffee consumed, the higher the blood cholesterol levels, but it is of interest that the good cholesterol was not significantly affected.

Why aren't saunas and steam baths included in the program?

Unfortunately steam baths and saunas have been promoted as healthful measures to rid the body of dangerous toxins and as a relaxation method. The truth is they have not been included because they are downright dangerous, particularly for people with heart disease. The increased heat actually diverts much of the blood from the heart area to the skin, which is directly in contact with the heat source, in an attempt to cool the body. This causes a reduction of the blood to the heart muscle and other organs, so less oxygen and nutriments are circulated to them. Hence people with cardiovascular disease who have narrowed coronary arteries are at increased risk because of the possiblity of lack of oxygen to the heart muscle resulting in either angina pain or heart attack.

But doesn't the same hold true for people who exercise and become heated up?

Yes, and this is the reason for the precautions given in the chapter on exercise to wear the proper exercise clothes and on hot humid days to exercise when it is cooler, in the morning or after sundown. A hot shower will further divert blood from the heart to the skin, thereby increasing the risk. Therefore, always wait at least an hour after exercising before taking a shower.

Is it dangerous to use tranquilizers when exercising?

Highly dangerous! This is true in any situation in which you become over-heated, as with exercise, during saunas or steam baths, while sunning at the beach or working in a hot room. Tranquilizers exert an adverse effect on the temperature-regulating system of the brain, called the *hypothalamus*, causing the temperature of the body to rise to high levels. This is called *hyperthermia* and causes destructive effects on the brain, heart, kidneys and other organs, thereby leading to death.

What is the status of low cholesterol levels and cancer?

An apparent link between blood cholesterol levels below 180 and other diseases such as colon cancer was first reported by the Framingham study and others, but this association has been disproved by a new ten-year international collaborative group investigation consisting of 61,567 men of forty to sixty-nine years of age in eight countries. Scientists found an increased incidence of cancer deaths in the first year of the study, associated with low cholesterol levels, but this level decreased in later years, suggesting that undiagnosed cancer caused the low cholesterol levels, not the converse.

Is sex an acceptable heart-saving exercise?

No, because cardiac conditioning is dependent on a sustained rhythmic acceleration of the heart rate within a person's target zone. An exercise must be performed for a minimum of fifteen to twenty minutes to gain physiological benefits. According to Masters and Johnson in their book *Human Sexual Response*, there are four phases of the sexual response: the excitement phase associated with foreplay, the intromission plateau, orgasm and the resolution or recovery phase. The orgasm or third phase, which lasts only ten to fifteen seconds, marks the period of maximal activity characterized by a rapid heart rate, elevated blood pressure and hyperventilation. This is the phase in which the heart works the hardest. Hellerstein and Freedman reported in 1971 that the energy level during sexual intercourse in terms of oxygen demand to the heart was equivalent only to climbing two flights of stairs or taking a brisk walk. Therefore, the sex phase of maximum activity is only equal to a low-level brisk walk, which would fall well below a person's target zone, and it is only sustained for ten to fifteen seconds.

Is sex off limits for a person who has had a heart attack or who suffers from anginal pain?

Most people in this category can withstand the demands of sexual relations without undue strain. The major concern of most men following a heart attack is the fear of having another attack. This fear frequently exists as a source of undue anxiety and tension translated in terms of impotence, ejaculation disorders, loss of libido and the like. The average male who recovers after an uncomplicated heart attack has a maximum energy expenditure of eight to nine metabolic units (mets). The phase of maximum activity of the heart during intercourse (orgasm phase) is only five to six mets, which is far below the maximum energy level.

Are there any recommendations for post-heart-attack patients regarding sexual activity?

The following recommendations should be followed:

1. Have a cardiac exercise stress test before resuming sexual activities.
2. Avoid sex for two to three hours after a heavy meal, because the digestive process imposes an additional work load on the cardiovascular system.
3. Pay heed to Dr. Sam Fox III's prescription for men regarding sex: It should be performed "with a mature approach orchestrated à la Debussy rather than Wagner." Further, Dr. Fox indicated that women "are not as impressed with the athletic prowess of a partner as many men seem to think. Ease up on the throttle and work on the technique."
4. If you experience any pain during sex, consult your physician. It is very common for a patient to take nitroglycerin or a long-acting medication before engaging in sexual activity. This will allow him or her to perform the sexual act by eliminating the anticipation of pain and allow the person to concentrate on lovemaking and not on the heart condition.

Many experts say that measures to fight heart disease should begin in childhood. Why? Children don't have heart attacks.
Medical evidence indicates that the accumulation of fatty substances—the precursors of heart disease—begin in childhood but take their toll in adulthood. There is much evidence that preventive measures instituted during early childhood may prevent heart disease.

What measures in particular should be instituted during childhood in an attempt to prevent coronary heart disease?
1. Periodic examinations to identify risk factors such as high blood pressure, elevated cholesterol and triglycerides, obesity and diabetes.
2. Apply the Heart-Saving Menu Plan so that it becomes an automatic way of life in the home. This is the most fruitful time in a person's life to enact such changes.
3. Avoid salt in a baby's food. Fortunately, in the mid-70s manufacturers agreed to stop adding salt to baby foods. Avoid salt whenever possible in all food ingested. Remove the salt shaker from the table.
4. Avoid obesity by establishing appropriate dietary habits in the home. Also set limits on candies and other desserts.
5. Promote regular physical activities as running, handball, basketball, jumping rope, swimming, tennis and so on. Set a limit on the time allowed to watch television. Many experts feel that much of the physical deterioration in teenagers is the result of watching too much television at the expense of physical activity.
6. Educate your child about the dangers of smoking. Insist on education programs in the school as well.

Can I substitute transcendental meditation for stress-control exercises?
Yes, you can substitute transcendental meditation for any meditation procedure in the stress-control program.

Is lecithin useful in reducing blood cholesterol levels?
Don't waste your money, because the cholesterol-lowering effect of lecithin is so minimal that it is worthless. It is a chemical compound called a phospholipid extracted from soybeans and used in candy, bread and drugs. It is found in animal tissues, including brain, nerve, liver, semen, egg yolk, bile, blood and cell membranes.

Are career women at greater risk of having a heart attack?
Yes. In recent years more women are claiming a role in the professional world. They are suffering the slings and arrows of corporate tensions,

assuming responsibility for large budgets and large staffs, eating high-fat meals on expense accounts and the like. Therefore, there has been a significant increase in the number of heart attacks among women. This was graphically pointed out in the *American Journal of Public Health* following an eight-year study concerning the incidence of coronary artery disease by employment status among men and women between forty-five and sixty-four years of age. In this study housewives had about 36 percent of the number of cases of coronary artery disease when compared to men, while working women had 54 percent. As more women enter the business world, the incidence will unquestionably rise further.

Is there such a thing as a silent heart attack?

Yes, and they are more common than you think. The Framingham study recently revealed that out of 259 heart attacks documented by an electrocardiogram, 20 percent of the victims were unaware they had had a heart attack. At the Office of the Medical Examiner in Rockland County, New York, autopsies are performed on all individuals who die suddenly without a significant history of heart disease. Yet we have found in an ongoing study that over 65 percent of them showed evidence at autopsy of having had a previous heart attack. A careful history may elicit an incident of vague pain, a bout of "indigestion," an attack of cold sweats or no symptoms at all. This information indicates that everyone over forty should have periodic electrocardiograms to identify the silent heart attack victim, so that appropriate preventive measures may be taken.

Once I stop smoking, can I take a cigarette now and then?

No, the ex-smoker must avoid a cigarette at all costs, in much the same way that an alcoholic on the wagon must never take another drink. This is because the nicotine tolerance appears to be permanent, and the ex-smoker may be hooked again even several years later.

What is passive smoking?

This refers not to smoking in the usual sense of the word but to inhaling smoke in the atmosphere resulting from cigarette smoke that does not pass through the cigarette and smoke that is exhaled by smokers. The first type of smoke, known as sidestream smoke, contains a higher concentration of tar, nicotine and noxious gases than the exhaled smoke.

Are children affected by passive smoking?

Statistically children have twice the incidence of pneumonia or bronchitis during the first year of life in homes where people smoke as compared to children who live in homes where there is no smoking.

How long does it take for a smoker's health profile to reach that of a nonsmoker?

If the habitual smoker stops before there is damage to the heart and lungs, it will take about ten years to reduce the risk of heart attack and ten to fifteen years to reduce the risk of lung cancer to that of the nonsmoker. The mortality risk also drops to that of the nonsmoker in ten to fifteen years.

If nicotine is a poison, why doesn't it kill a heavy smoker?

It takes about 60 milligrams (about $\frac{1}{1000}$ of an ounce) of nicotine to kill the average person by paralyzing the breathing mechanism. Smokers inhale very tiny amounts, and this is rapidly metabolized and eliminated by the body. Nicotine also causes an increase in blood pressure and pulse rate.

Chapter Ten

After 14 Days

He who hath good health is young.
—Francis Bacon

I hope that the foregoing chapters have answered your questions about heart attacks and have motivated you to begin the 14-day program to prevent heart disease. Remember, you must have patience and motivation to succeed, since our current habits have been ingrained for years and can't be changed overnight. In this chapter I am going to tell you how to maintain the new routine beyond fourteen days, so that you can *permanently* change your life.

YOUR EXERCISE PLAN AFTER 14 DAYS

Walking

WEEK 3 TO WEEK 12

Increase the time for brisk walking 2 minutes each week. Remember to do warm-up and cool-down exercises prior to and after every brisk walk. During the twelfth week you will be doing the brisk walk for 29 minutes. Do your exercise program for a minimum of four days each week.

AFTER WEEK 12

From the thirteenth week on, perform the brisk walk for 30 minutes. Remember to check your pulse periodically to see if you are exercising within your target zone.

Jogging

WEEK 3 TO WEEK 15

A 5-minute warm-up and a 5-minute cool-down exercise must be done prior to and after jogging, using the following procedure:

Before Jogging

5 minutes	group 2, warm-up cool-down exercises every day prior to jogging

After Jogging

3 minutes	walk slowly
2 minutes	group 2, warm-up cool-down exercises

Jogging Program

Week 3	walk 5 minutes, jog 3 minutes
	walk 5 minutes, jog 3 minutes
Weeks 4 and 5	walk 4 minutes, jog 5 minutes
	walk 4 minutes, jog 5 minutes
Week 6	walk 4 minutes, jog 6 minutes
	walk 4 minutes, jog 6 minutes
Week 7	walk 4 minutes, jog 7 minutes
	walk 4 minutes, jog 7 minutes
Week 8	walk 4 minutes, jog 6 minutes
	walk 4 minutes, jog 8 minutes
Week 9	walk 4 minutes, jog 9 minutes
Week 10	walk 4 minutes, jog 13 minutes
Week 11	walk 4 minutes, jog 15 minutes
Week 12	walk 4 minutes, jog 17 minutes
Week 13	walk 2 minutes, slow jog 2 minutes, jog 17 minutes
Week 14	walk 1 minute, slow jog 3 minutes, jog 17 minutes
Week 15	jog slowly 3 minutes, jog 17 minutes

AFTER WEEK 16

Continue jogging at least four days each week, using the program of Week 15.

Cycling

WEEK 3

5 minutes	group 2, warm-up cool-down exercises
2 minutes	cycle at 60 cycles a minute without tension
12 minutes	cycle at 60 cycles a minute, slowly increasing the tension and checking your pulse until you reach the lower limit of your target zone
5 minutes	group 2, warm-up cool-down exercises

WEEK 4

5 minutes	group 2, warm-up cool-down exercises
2 minutes	cycle at 60 cycles a minute without tension
14 minutes	cycle at 60 cycles a minute with tension regulated to your target zone
5 minutes	group 2, warm-up cool-down exercises

WEEK 5

5 minutes	group 2, warm-up cool-down exercises
2 minutes	cycle at 60 cycles a minute without tension
16 minutes	cycle at 60 cycles a minute with tension regulated to your target zone
5 minutes	group 2, warm-up cool-down exercises

WEEK 6

5 minutes	group 2, warm-up cool-down exercises
2 minutes	cycle at 60 cycles a minute without tension
18 minutes	cycle at 60 cycles a minute with tension regulated to your target zone
5 minutes	group 2, warm-up cool-down exercises

AFTER WEEK 6

5 minutes	group 2, warm-up cool-down exercises
2 minutes	cycle at 60 cycles a minute without tension
20 minutes	cycle at 60 cycles a minute with tension regulated to your target zone
5 minutes	group 2, warm-up cool-down exercises

Jumping Rope

After 14 Days
5 minutes   group 2, warm-up cool-down exercises

Use the same regimen as for days 10 to 14, except add 10 jumps to each jumping period every week until you reach 100 jumps in each jumping period, for a total of 300 jumps each day (week 9).

Swimming—Low Gear

WEEK 3 TO WEEK 6
Follow the same routine, except swim two pool lengths each time for the first week, then increase by one pool length each week until you are swimming five pool lengths each time. You should begin checking your pulse so that you are swimming at the lower level of your target zone.

AFTER WEEK 7
Same as for weeks 3 to 6, but swim 4 minutes right in your target zone, then ease off with a lazy breast or side stroke until you feel recovered, then continue with 2 additional minutes each week until you reach the level of 10 minutes.

Swimming—High Gear

WEEK 3
Do the same as for the low-gear program, except the lap swimming, which should be done continuously for 10 minutes with pulse monitoring to stay within your target zone. If you exceed your target zone or you feel winded, ease off by doing a lazy breast or side stroke until you feel recovered, then continue.

AFTER WEEK 4
Do the same as for week 3, except increase the lap time by 2 minutes each week until you reach 20 minutes.

Trampoline
The walking-type program and the jogging-type program should be increased, using the format of the regular walking and jogging programs.

The mixed-routine trampoline program given in the 14-Day Heart-Saving Exercise Plan in chapter 2 should be continued as is. The maximum work-out time could be slowly advanced over several weeks to 30 minutes.

YOUR DIET PLAN AFTER 14 DAYS

How to Modify Your Own Recipes

1. Critically evaluate your recipes, using all the principles you have learned thus far. Go through the list of food substitutes on pages 65–67 and determine if substitution appears practical for a particular recipe. If the recipe contains several components that would require substitution, or if it would require replacing large amounts of a saturated fat or high-cholesterol food, discard it. An example of this is croissants, which can be made with soft margarine, but the amount of fat required is prohibitive.
2. If the recipe calls for butter, substitute a smaller amount of soft margarine, an acceptable vegetable oil, a mixture of both, or the poly spread (see recipe section in Appendix). Try different oils, as some may leave an aftertaste in some recipes. For example, corn oil leaves a corn aftertaste in the poly "ice cream" and poly "whipped cream" recipes. Try substituting smaller and smaller amounts until you achieve the desirable effect with the least amount possible.
3. Strip the amount of sodium in your recipes. If a recipe calls for a teaspoon of salt, try eliminating it completely, cutting down on the amount, substituting a sodium/potassium salt, or using some other flavoring, such as lemon juice or one of the seasonings suggested on page 110.
4. When sugar is required, cut down on the amount, use a sugar substitute, a mixture of sugar and sugar substitute, honey or a fruit sugar.
5. If a recipe calls for eggs, separate the yolks and substitute about 6 whites and 1 yolk for 3 whole eggs. This is even true when preparing an eggnog. In some recipes you can merely substitute egg whites and you will not be able to tell the difference. Try egg substitutes whenever possible. Also remember that whenever you prepare a recipe, figure the number of people that will be eating it and divide by that number. This will greatly reduce the cholesterol content that each person ingests.
6. Whole milk or cream can usually be replaced by skim milk to which

nonfat milk solids are added. In some instances, you can add a small amount of oil to the skim milk. A white sauce by heating oil, mixing in the flour, and adding skim milk and stirring until thick.

7. When a recipe requires chocolate, try a small amount of cocoa or carob. Carob is made from the dried pods and seeds of the carob tree. The taste is very delicate and similar to chocolate and cocoa. A teaspoon contains only about 7 calories and is high in vitamins and minerals.

Make a Gradual Change in Your Dietary Life-style

Our dietary habits have been deeply ingrained over a lifetime. Change requires a slow transition over many months, with constant practice and conditioning to create a new dietary life-style. This should be done gradually and in stages, so that everything is done in an automatic manner.

STAGE ONE: THE FIRST SIX MONTHS

The change should be implemented in a gradual manner over this period. For example, at the beginning of this stage trim all the visible fats on meats; cook at the lower temperatures indicated; substitute 2-percent milk for whole milk at some of the meals, then gradually replace more and more of the whole milk over several months until no more of the latter is used. Substitute soft margarine for butter on the table and in cooking, cut out frying, put less and less salt in food over several months, and begin reducing red meat by 1 meal every few weeks until it is served at only one meal each week. Start eating one fish meal and one chicken meal each week and increase slowly so that after several weeks you are eating two fish meals, two chicken meals, two no-meat meals and one red-meat meal. Begin using in a few of your recipes some of the foods listed under Foods and Acceptable Substitutes on page 65, and gradually substitute more of them over the weeks until you are doing it as a matter of course. At the same time try some of the recipes included in the Appendix. Add unprocessed bran, nuts, sunflower seeds and the like to salads, meat loafs, cereals and stews. Serve fruits during meals, after meals and in the evenings. Try low-fat low-cholesterol cheeses. Slowly implement the various ways to reduce saturated fats, total fats, cholesterol and sugar in your diet, and to increase fiber and starch as you were instructed in chapter 3. When you go shopping, read labels, and stop buying foods high in cholesterol, saturated fats, sodium and sugar.

STAGE TWO: SIX MONTHS AND GRADUALLY THEREAFTER FOR LIFE

When you complete Stage One, you will have drastically reduced the amount of saturated fat, cholesterol, sugar and sodium in your diet. Remember, in doing this you will automatically be reducing calories as well. Stage Two stresses a continuation of the routine established in Stage One and further emphasizes a reduction in the intake of food items that are high in fats and cholesterol. This is important to ensure achieving the objectives of the 14-Day Heart-Saving Diet Plan.

Egg yolks and poultry skin must have been completely eliminated from the diet at this stage. A gradual reduction of meat intake must be instituted over several months until no more than 6 to 9 ounces of meat is eaten each day, depending on a person's caloric intake. This amount is given for each calorie level in the Low-Fat Low-Cholesterol Weight Reduction Plan in Appendix A. Note that a meat exchange is equal to 3 ounces of meat. Therefore 6 to 9 ounces of meat is equal to 3 meat exchanges. Determine your caloric level so you will know how much meat you are allotted (see p. 171). For example, if your caloric level is 2200 calories each day, you are allowed the maximum of 9 ounces of meat.

More and more foods high in complex carbohydrates and fiber must be incorporated into your diet (grains, vegetables, nuts, beans, fruits, cereals, etc.).

YOUR QUIT-SMOKING PLAN AFTER 14 DAYS

Congratulations! Now that you have quit smoking, it is important that you stay quit. Remember, the longer you stay away from a smoke, the easier it will be to resist. Study the following tips.

Tips to Help You Stay Quit

- Avoid smokers who may want to see you continue smoking.
- If possible, try quitting with a friend and keep in touch with each other daily.
- Let other people know you are quitting. This is a way to put pressure on yourself to quit.
- Leave the table and brush your teeth after each meal.
- Make a Reward-Yourself List of items you would like to have, like a new fishing rod, TV set, bowling ball, tape deck, carpenter tools. Estimate the price of each in terms of the cost of a week's supply of cigarettes and earmark this money in a special container.

- Make life changes so that you spend more time in libraries, buses, theaters, etc. during the first weeks of quitting.
- Plan a party to celebrate your first month off cigarettes and a big party to celebrate six months off.
- Save books, crossword puzzles, quizzes, etc. to do during work breaks.
- Try to help others quit smoking, particularly your spouse, your family and your friends. Call your American Cancer Society unit and American Heart Association chapter and volunteer your services to help new ex-smokers stay quit.
- Try going to bed early and rising a half-hour earlier than usual to avoid hurrying through breakfast and rushing to work.
- If you were a "kitchen smoker" in the morning, volunteer your services to schools or nonprofit organizations to get you out of the house.
- After you have quit, never face the confusion of craving a cigarette alone. Find someone you can call or visit at this critical time.
- Visit your dentist after you quit and begin your new life with bright, white teeth. Try using lemon juice to remove the tobacco stains from your fingers.
- Get out of your old habits. Seek new activities or perform old activities in new ways. Don't rely on the old ways of solving problems. Do things differently.

YOUR BLOOD PRESSURE CONTROL PLAN AFTER 14 DAYS

You are now on your way to blood pressure control. You must never lose track of the fact that blood pressure control is a lifelong commitment requiring constant surveillance of your blood pressure, body weight, sodium intake, physical activity level and ancillary factors. Place the following first four recommendations on your calendar and faithfully adhere to them.

1. Weigh yourself once each week. If you have gained more than 2 pounds, begin weight reduction according to the Low-Fat Low-Cholesterol Weight Reduction Plan in Appendix A. If you note that your weight gain occurs frequently, record everything you eat for one week and your daily weight in a diary and analyze where you went wrong. This will help you make the necessary adjustments to prevent this from happening.

2. Take your blood pressure once each week and record the readings in your diary in chart form. This will serve as a record so that you can see how you are doing with your program, and your doctor can observe your progress.
3. Exercise a miniumum of four days each week according to the Exercise Plan After 14 Days beginning on page 159, and try to do it at the same time each day.
4. Perform your meditation procedure (chapter 6) at the same time every day.
5. Keep up the habit of reading labels to determine the sodium content of foods.
6. Follow the Quit-Smoking Plan After 14 Days on page 165 if you quit smoking recently.
7. Continue to avoid oral contraceptives.

YOUR STRESS MODIFICATION PLAN AFTER 14 DAYS

In the fourteen-day period you have learned the basic tools to assist you in combatting a multitude of the most commonly encountered stressful situations and experiences. You must practice and use the various relaxation procedures regularly, do the meditation technique every day without fail, continually work on modifying your undesirable behavior patterns, evaluate your time management and continue taking notes regarding your stressful experiences and self-contracts.

YOUR DIABETES CONTROL PLAN AFTER 14 DAYS

Successful diabetes control largely depends on a lifetime commitment to weight control; strict adherence to a low-fat, low-cholesterol, high-fiber diet; regular exercise; control of high blood pressure; proper care of infections; and change in your habits so that these are done automatically. The first two recommendations that follow should be placed prominently on your calendar so they can be done without fail.

1. Exercise a minumum of four days each week according to the Exercise Plan After 14 Days on page 159 and try to do it at the same time each day.

2. Continue with the Diet Plan After 14 Days that follows.
3. Continue using at least 50 grams of fiber each day.
4. Avoid oral contraceptives.

I hope the end of this book will be the beginning of a new life-style that will promote your cardiovascular health, afford you a sense of well-being and add years to your life. If you stick with it, the dividends you reap will be legion. Good Luck.

APPENDIXES

Your body is the baggage you must carry through life. The more excess baggage, the shorter the trip.

Arnold H. Glasow

Low-Fat Low-Cholesterol

Weight Reduction Plan

The Low-Fat Low-Cholesterol Weight Reduction Plan will lower your total blood cholesterol, your bad cholesterol and your triglycerides. At the same time it will raise your good cholesterol and reduce dietary sodium and sugar. This low-fat low-cholesterol diet plan employs a food-exchange technique that is easy to use and adds variety to your meals.

Menus from 1000 calories to 2400 calories have been developed to provide you with well-balanced meals. Use the following procedure to determine the calorie level you must use in order to lose about 2 pounds each week, and then select the corresponding menu plan.

Determining Your Calorie Level to Lose Weight

1. Determine the weight you should be for your height and build from the chart on page 174 (your goal). _____ pounds
2. What is your present weight? _____ pounds
3. Multiply your present weight by one of the following to determine your present caloric intake.

   If you do very hard labor, multiply by 20. _____ cals
   If you do hard labor, multiply by 18. _____ cals
   If you do moderately active work, multiply by 16. _____ cals
   If your work is sedentary, multiply by 13. _____ cals

4. Subtract 1200 calories from your present caloric intake to lose 2 pounds each week. (There is a loss of 1 additional pound for every 600 calories subtracted each day.)

For example, a secretary, 5 feet 6 inches tall, of medium build and weighing 185 pounds, desires to reach her average weight. Her weight on the table averages

137 pounds (her goal). She would multiply 185 lbs. $\times$ 13 to get 2405 calories. This is her present caloric intake (the number of calories needed to keep her weight constant at 185 lbs.).

To lose 2 pounds each week—2405 minus 1200 = 1205 calories. She would select the 1200-calorie Low-Fat Low-Cholesterol Menu using the exchanges for the 1200-calorie diet listed on the Exchange Chart.

Daily Menu Plans with

Good Exchanges

The exchange system of menu planning has been adopted because of its great success in withstanding the test of time in the planning of menus for diabetics. There are six groups of food exchanges: lean meat exchanges, skim milk exchanges, bread exchanges, vegetable exchanges, fruit exchanges and vegetable fat exchanges. All the food items in these menus are placed in one of these groups for your selection. Regard each exchange as a serving. All exchanges in the same group can be exchanged for each other, but food exchanges from one group can *not* be exchanged from any other group, because the nutrient compositions differ.

The menu plans have been divided into three meals and three between-meal snacks: mid-morning, mid-afternoon and evening. The total calories from fat in the menus vary between 22 and 27 percent, being greater than 25 percent in plans above 1600 calories. The cholesterol content ranges from 80 milligrams in the 1000-calorie menu to well below 250 in the 2400-calorie menu, and the polyunsaturates are well below the 10-percent range.

After you determine your calorie-intake level according to the instructions on pages 171 to 172, select the number of exchanges indicated on the following chart and formulate a menu plan using the corresponding sample menu as a guide.

EXCHANGE CHART
[Select Your Menu]

Calories	1000	1200	1400	1600	1800	2000	2400
meat exchanges	1.0	1.5	2.0	2.5	3.0	3.0	3.0
skim milk exchanges	1.0	1.0	1.0	1.0	1.0	1.0	1.0
bread exchanges	4.0	6.0	7.0	8.0	9.0	11.0	14.0
vegetable exchanges	3.0	3.0	3.0	3.0	3.0	3.0	4.0
fruit exchanges	6.0	7.0	7.0	7.0	7.0	8.0	10.0
fat exchanges	3.0	3.0	3.0	4.0	5.0	6.0	8.0

1983 Metropolitan Height and Weight Tables
for Men and Women According to Frame, Ages 25–59

		Weight in Pounds (in Indoor Clothing)*		
Height **(In Shoes)†**		**Small** **Frame**	**Medium** **Frame**	**Large** **Frame**
FEET	INCHES		MEN	
5	2	128–134	131–141	138–150
5	3	130–136	133–143	140–153
5	4	132–138	135–145	142–156
5	5	134–140	137–148	144–160
5	6	136–142	139–151	146–164
5	7	138–145	142–154	149–168
5	8	140–148	145–157	152–172
5	9	142–151	148–160	155–176
5	10	144–154	151–163	158–180
5	11	146–157	154–166	161–184
6	0	149–160	157–170	164–188
6	1	152–164	160–174	168–192
6	2	155–168	164–178	172–197
6	3	158–172	167–182	176–202
6	4	162–176	171–187	181–207
			WOMEN	
4	10	102–111	109–121	118–131
4	11	103–113	111–123	120–134
5	0	104–115	113–126	122–137
5	1	106–118	115–129	125–140
5	2	108–121	118–132	128–143
5	3	111–124	121–135	131–147
5	4	114–127	124–138	134–151
5	5	117–130	127–141	137–155
5	6	120–133	130–144	140–159
5	7	123–136	133–147	143–163
5	8	126–139	136–150	146–167
5	9	129–142	139–153	149–170
5	10	132–145	142–156	152–173
5	11	135–148	145–159	155–176
6	0	138–151	148–162	158–179

NOTE: Reprinted courtesy of Metropolitan Life Insurance Company. Source of basic data: *Build Study*, 1979, Society of Actuaries and Association of Life Insurance Medical Directors of America, 1980. Copyright 1983 Metropolitan Life Insurance Company.

*Indoor clothing weighing 5 pounds for men and 3 pounds for women
†Shoes with 1-inch heels

How to Determine Your Body Frame by Elbow Breadth

To make a simple approximation of your frame size:

Extend your arm and bend the forearm upwards at a 90-degree angle. Keep the fingers straight and turn the inside of your wrists toward the body. Place the thumb and index finger of your other hand on the two prominent bones on either side of your elbow. Measure the space between your fingers against a ruler or a tape measure. (For the most accurate measurement, have you physician measure your elbow breadth with calipers.) Compare this measurement with the measurements shown below.

These tables list the elbow measurements for men and women of medium frame at various heights. Measurements lower than those listed indicate that you have a small frame while higher measurements indicate a large frame.

MEN

Height (In 1-inch Heels)	Elbow Breadth (Inches)	Height (In 2.5-cm. Heels)	Elbow Breadth (Centimeters)
5'2"–5"3"	2½"–2⅞"	158–161	6.4–7.2
5'4"–5'7"	2⅝"–2⅞"	162–171	6.7–7.4
5'8"–5'11"	2¾–3	172–181	6.9–7.6
6'0"–6'3"	2¾"–3⅛"	182–191	7.1–7.8
6'4"	2⅞"–3¼"	192–193	7.4–8.1

WOMEN

Height (In 1-inch Heels)	Elbow Breadth (Inches)	Height (In 2.5-cm Heels)	Elbow Breadth (Centimeters)
4'10"–4'11"	2¼"–2½"	148–151	5.6–6.4
5'0"–5'3"	2¼"–2½"	152–161	5.8–6.5
5'4"–5'7"	2⅜"–2⅝"	162–171	5.9–6.6
5'8"–5'11"	2⅜"–2⅝"	172–181	6.1–6.8
6'0"	2½"–2¾"	182–183	6.2–6.9

NOTE: Reprinted courtesy of Metropolitan Life Insurance Company.

Source of basic data: Data tape. HANES I—Anthropometry, goniometry, skeletal age, bone density, and cortical thickness, ages 1–74. National Health and Nutrition Examination Survey. 1971–75, National Center for Health Statistics.

Copyright 1983 Metropolitan Life Insurance Company.

SAMPLE MENU: 1000 Calories

Meal	Food	Exchange
Breakfast	1 cup grapefruit juice	2 fruit
	2 slices white bread	2 bread
	1 tsp. margarine	1 fat
	1 cup black coffee or tea	free
Mid-A.M. Snack	1 apple	1 fruit
	1 cup black coffee or tea	free
Lunch	1 cup lettuce for salad	1 vegetable
	1 tsp. French dressing	1 fat
	1 pear	1 fruit
	1 cup black coffee, tea or	free
	1 bottle sugar-free beverage	free
Mid-P.M. Snack	1 cup beef broth, fat free	free
	1 cup black coffee or tea	free
Dinner	3 ounces chicken	1 meat
	½ cup rice	1 bread
	1 tbsp. fat-free gravy	1 free
	½ cup carrots	1 vegetable
	½ cup peas	1 vegetable
	½ cup fruit cocktail	1 fruit
	1 cup black coffee or tea	free
Evening Snack	1 cup skim milk	1 milk
	1⅓ cup Jell-O	1 bread
	1 cup coffee or tea	1 free

SAMPLE MENU: 1400 Calories

Meal	Food	Exchange
Breakfast	1 cup orange juice	2 fruit
	1 cup cooked cereal	2 bread
	½ cup skim milk	½ milk
	1 cup black coffee or tea	free

Mid-A.M. Snack	1 hard roll	1 bread
	1 banana	2 fruit
	1 cup black coffee or tea	free
Lunch	3 ounces tuna fish	1 meat
	1 tsp. mayonnaise	1 fat
	2 slices white bread	2 bread
	1 cup black coffee, tea or	free
	1 bottle sugar-free beverage	free
Mid-P.M. Snack	1 peach	1 fruit
	1 cup black coffee or tea	free
Dinner	3 ounces veal	1 meat
	½ cup macaroni	1 bread
	1 tbsp. fat-free gravy	1 free
	½ cup broccoli	1 vegetable
	1 cup tomatoes	2 vegetable
	½ honeydew melon	2 fruit
	1 cup black coffee or tea	free
Evening Snack	½ cup skim milk	½ milk
	½ English muffin	1 bread
	1 tsp. margarine	1 fat
	1 cup black coffee or tea	1 free

SAMPLE MENU: 1600 Calories

Meal	**Food**	**Exchange**
Breakfast	1 cup orange juice	2 fruit
	2 slices whole wheat toast	2 bread
	1 tsp. margarine	1 fat
	1 cup black coffee or tea	free
Mid-A.M. Snack	2 honey graham crakers	1 bread
	1 cup black coffee or tea	free
Lunch	1 peanut butter sandwich	2 bread
	made with 2 tsp. peanut butter	2 fat
	1 apple	1 fruit
	1 cup black coffee, tea or	free
	1 bottle sugar-free beverage	free

Mid-P.M.	1 cup beef broth, fat free	free
Snack	1 banana	2 fruit
Dinner	7½ ounces roast beef	2½ meat
	½ cup mashed potatoes	1 bread
	½ cup green beans	1 vegetable
	1 cup lettuce, for salad	2 vegetable
	(no restriction on amount)	
	1 tbsp. French dressing	1 fat
	½ cup applesauce	1 fruit
	1 3-inch cube angel-food cake	1 bread
	1 cup black coffee or tea	free
Evening	¾ cup dry cereal	1 bread
Snack	1 cup skim milk with	1 milk
	artificial sweetener	free
	1 orange	1 fruit

SAMPLE MENU: 1800 Calories

Meal	**Food**	**Exchange**
Breakfast	1 cup orange juice	2 fruit
	2 slices whole wheat bread	2 bread
	1 tsp. margarine	1 fat
	½ grapefruit	1 fruit
	1 cup black coffee or tea	free
Mid-A.M.	1 English muffin	2 bread
Snack	1 tsp. margarine	1 fat
	1 cup black coffee or tea	free
Lunch	3 ounces chicken salad	1 meat
	1 tsp. mayonnaise	1 fat
	2 slices white bread	2 bread
	¼ cantaloupe	1 fruit
	1 cup black coffee, tea or	free
	1 bottle sugar-free beverage	free
Mid-P.M.	2 graham crackers	1 bread
Snack	1 cup black coffee or tea	free

Dinner	6 ounces salmon	2 meat
	1 cup rice	2 bread
	1 tbsp. fat-free gravy	1 free
	½ cup cauliflower	1 vegetable
	½ cup mushrooms	1 vegetable
	cup lettuce, for salad	1 vegetable
	½ tbsp. Italian dressing	1 fat
	½ cup applesauce	1 fruit
	1 cup black coffee or tea	free
Evening	1 cup skim milk	1 milk
Snack	1 cup blueberries	2 fruit
	1 cup black coffee or tea	1 free

FOOD EXCHANGES

Lean Meat, Poultry, Fish Exchanges

Limit your choice to very lean meat; avoid meat cuts marbled or streaked with fat. Trim off all fat. Remove skin from poultry before eating. *Avoid fried foods* except those fried in the fat allowed in this diet.

Keep the following ideas in mind when you estimate your *three-ounce* portion:

1. When raw meat, poultry, or fish is cooked, its weight becomes less by virtue of loss of water during the cooking process. Without bone four ounces raw weight becomes approximately three ounces cooked.
2. One-half large breast of chicken is approximately three ounces cooked, edible portion; one thigh plus one drumstick is approximately three ounces cooked, edible portion.
3. Meat, poultry, or fish cooked, and then flaked or chopped, may be measured in a cup; three-fourths cup is approximately three ounces.

Note: Three ounces of these foods is considered one portion, or approximately 177 Calories.

Beef	**Use**	**Avoid**
Beef round	Rump roast	Fatty meat
Round roast	Sirloin tip	Organ meats
Ground round	Tenderloin	Meats canned or frozen
Corned beef round	Dried beef	in gravy
Smoked beef		Fried meat other than
		those fried in allowed
Veal		fat
Arm steak		Canned meat products
Sirloin roast and steak		Luncheon meat, cold
Rump roast		cuts
Loin chop		Hamburger

Use		Avoid
Lamb		Wieners (frankfurters)
Roast leg		Sausages
Loin chop		Spare ribs
Pork		Pork butt
Sirloin roast	Tenderloin	Picnic shoulder
Center-cut loin chop	Lean ham	Pork steak
Center-cut ham steak	Canadian bacon	Bacon
Poultry		Veal cutlets
Chicken	Cornish hen	Lamb blade chops
Turkey	Game birds	Corned beef brisket
Fish		All poultry skin
Bass	Halibut	Goose
Brook trout	Perch	Duck
Catfish	Pike	Caviar
Cod	Salmon	Crabs
Crappie (sunfish)	Swordfish	Shrimp
Flounder	Waterpacked tuna	Lobster
Haddock	Whitefish	
Sardines	Trout	
Mackerel	Herring	
Clams	Scallops	
Oysters		

NOTE: Food Exchange Lists from "A Maximal Approach to the Dietary Treatment of the Hyperlipidemias," taken from *A Low Cholesterol Diet Manual* with permission of W. E. Connor, M.D. (Iowa City: University of Iowa Press, 1968).

Fat Exchanges

Complete hydrogenation generally produces saturated or "hard" fat which should be avoided. Soft margarines, soft "diet" margarines and some vegetable shortenings are satisfactory, as are certain stick margarines because they are only slightly hydrogenated. To be acceptable, margarines and shortenings should contain no animal fat, and labels should show a predominance of polyunsaturated fat which has not been hardened. Suitable liquid vegetable oils which contain a considerable amount of polyunsaturated fat are: corn, cottonseed, soybean, safflower, sunflower, and peanut. (Olive oil is largely monounsaturated and may be used occasionally.)

Note: Each of the following in the amount listed is considered one Fat Exchange (approximately 45 Calories).

Use	Avoid
1 teaspoon unsalted vegetable oil margarine or 2 teaspoons low-calorie unsalted margarine	Butter and products made with butter Margarines and shortenings which are heavily hydrogenated or salted
1 teaspoon vegetable oil	Lard, suet, bacon fat, meat drippings

Use	**Avoid**
1 teaspoon vegetable shortening	Coconut oil, palm oil, palm kernel oil,
2 teaspoons peanut butter	and products containing these fats[2]
1 tablespoon French or Italian	Products such as cookies and
dressing[1]	crackers which contain animal fat
1 tablespoon coarsely chopped nuts	Mayonnaise or other dressings and
5 small olives	sauces which contain egg yolk,
⅛ avocado	whole milk, or animal fat
1½ tablespoons soybean bacon bits	Chocolate
	Coconut

[1] Limited amounts of low-calorie dressings made without egg yolk may be used without exchanging.

[2] Whipped toppings (dry mix or fully prepared) contain small amounts of coconut oil or other saturated fat. Their use must be limited to 2 tablespoons prepared and this amount is to be considered ½ Fat Exchange.

Skim Milk Exchanges

Skim milk is equal in nutritive value to whole milk except for fat and fat-soluble vitamins. These vitamins are supplied in this diet by fortified margarine and fortified skim milk of less than 0.5% butterfat content.

Egg whites and dried or rinsed cottage cheese are valuable sources of animal protein and should be used freely if calories are not restricted.

Other skim milk cheeses, such as sapsago, are allowed, and strictly limited amounts of Parmesan may be used for flavoring (a maximum of 1 tablespoon is allowed).

Note: Each of the following foods in the amount listed is considered one Skim Milk Exchange (approximately 110 Calories).

Use	**Avoid**
¾ cup low-fat yogurt	Whole milk in any form: fluid, dried,
	condensed, or evaporated
1 cup skim milk	Cheeses, other than those allowed
1 cup fortified skim milk of 0.5%	Cream in any form, sweet or sour
butterfat or less	
1 cup buttermilk if made from skim	Egg yolk or whole egg, and products
milk	containing either
1 cup buttermilk if made from skim	Filled milks which contain coconut oil
milk	
½ cup undiluted evaporated skim milk	
⅓ cup instant dry non-fat milk powder	
½ cup dried or rinsed cottage cheese[1]	
4 large egg whites	
Skim milk cheeses[2]	

[1] Place large-curd creamed cottage cheese in a colander and rinse thoroughly under cold water to remove the cream.

[2] The skim milk cheeses made with added "acceptable" vegetable fat may be used and exchanged as follows: 1 ounce of cheese for 1 Skim Milk Exchange plus 2 Fat Exchanges.

Bread Exchanges

Note: Each of the following in the amount listed is considered one Bread Exchange (approximately 70 Calories).

Use	Avoid
BREADS, CRACKERS, SHERBETS, ETC.	Commercially baked goods (other than bread)
½ cup cooked cereal	Hot roll mix
¾ cup dry ready-to-eat cereal	Prepared cake mix
¼ cup Grape-Nuts	Flavored crackers
1 slice bread (enriched white, Vienna, whole wheat or rye)	Cheese crackers
1 small hard roll	Ice cream, ice milk, frozen desserts containing coconut oil
1 hamburger bun (from package of 12)	Frozen breaded foods
2 graham cracker squares	Frozen French-fried potatoes
½ English muffin	Noodles
4 rectangles melba toast	Brown and serve rolls
3 soda crackers	Potato chips, corn chips
5 saltines	Pork and beans
1½" cube angel food cake	Sweet rolls
2½ tablespoons flour	Dinner rolls
15 small pretzel sticks	
2 tablespoons wheat germ	
¼ cup sherbet	
⅓ cup Jell-O	
½ cup cooked spaghetti, macaroni or rice	
1½ cups popcorn, popped (no added fat)	

Use

HIGH CARBOHYDRATE VEGETABLES (for other vegetables, see Vegetable Exchanges)

½ cup mashed potato or 2" potato
⅓ cup mashed sweet potato or yam
½ cup lima beans, cooked*
½ small sweet potato or yam
¼ cup baked beans without meat
½ cup dried beans (lima, navy, etc.)*
½ cup dried peas (split peas, etc.) or dried lentils*
⅓ cup corn or ½ medium ear

*These legumes are a valuable source of good-quality protein and should be included in the diet frequently.

Vegetable Exchanges

Because of their high-nutrient, low-calorie content, vegetables should generally be used freely and should rarely be limited to the indicated amounts.

Note: One-half cup of any vegetable cooked is equivalent to one Vegetable Exchange.

	Use	**Avoid**
Artichokes	Pumpkin	Deep-fat-fried
Asparagus	Romaine	vegetables
Bean sprouts	Rutabagas	Vegetables frozen in
Beets	Salsify	sauces and butter
Broccoli	Sauerkraut	Breaded vegetables
Brussels sprouts	Spinach	
Cabbage	Squash	
Carrots	Tomato juice	
Cauliflower	Tomatoes	
Celery	Turnips	
Chinese cabbage	Vegetable juice	
Eggplant	Wax beans	
Escarole		
Greenbeans	*Interesting Additions:*	
Greens	Chinese vegetables	
Lettuce	Garlic	
Mushrooms	Parsley	
Okra	Pimento	
Onions	Shallots	
Peas	Water chestnuts	
Peppers		

*Corn, lima beans, sweet potatoes, dried peas, dried beans, and lentils are listed under Bread Exchanges.

Use

Selected Soups*

Place cans of condensed soup in the refrigerator overnight. Remove fat accumulated at the top before heating. Prepare soups as directed. Use skim milk instead of whole milk where necessary. One serving is equivalent in calories to one Vegetable Exchange.

Campbell's (condensed)

Black bean	Chicken with rice
Chicken gumbo	Onion
Green pea	Vegetable beef
Cream of potato	Old-fashioned vegetable
Tomato	Vegetarian vegetable
Tomato rice	Chicken vegetable
Vegetable	

*Each serving contains less than 2 grams of fat.

Heinz (condensed)
Chicken gumbo
Cream of pea
Chicken vegetable

The following soups may be used without exchanging. (They contain no fat.)
Beef broth or consomme
Chicken broth or consomme

Fruit Exchanges

Fresh or sugarless frozen or sugarless canned fruits and juices are recommended in order to provide servings of reasonable sizes. However, on a diet of over 2000 Calories for a woman or over 2400 Calories for a man, sugar-sweetened canned or frozen fruits may be used.

Fresh Fruits and Fruit Juices
 Note: Each of the following in the amounts listed is considered one Fruit Exchange (approximately 40 Calories). These fruits are unsweetened, fresh, or dried; the juices are unsweetened fresh, frozen or canned.

Apple 1 small
Apricots 2 medium
Banana ½ small
Blackberries ½ cup
Blueberries ½ cup
Cantaloupe, diced or balls ½ cup
Cantaloupe (6" diameter) ¼ of whole
Cherries 10 large
Cranberries (artificially sweetened) 1 cup
Mixed fruit (cubes) ½ cup
Grapefruit ½ small
Grapes 12 medium
Honeydew melon (7" diameter) ⅛ whole
Orange 1 small
Peach 1 medium
Pear 1 small

Pineapple, cubed ½ cup
Plums 2 medium
Raspberries ½ cup
Strawberries 1 cup
Tangerine 1 large
Watermelon, diced or balls 1 cup
Apple juice or cider ⅓ cup
Apricot juice ½ cup
Grape juice ¼ cup
Grapefruit juice ½ cup
Orange juice ½ cup
Pineapple juice ⅓ cup
Prune juice ¼ cup

Rhubarb, if artificially sweetened, may be used freely

Avoid deep-fat-fried fruit and fruit fritters

Dried Fruits
 Note: Each of the following in the amount listed is considered one Fruit Exchange (approximately 40 Calories).

Apricots 3 large halves, uncooked or cooked without sugar
      1 half with 1 tablespoon juice, cooked and sweetened
Dates 2 medium
Figs 2 small or 1 large

Peaches   2 large halves, uncooked or cooked without sugar
3 small halves with juice, cooked and unsweetened
Prunes   2 medium uncooked or cooked without sugar
1 medium with 1 tablespoon juice, cooked and sweetened
1 large with juice, cooked, no sugar
Raisins   2 tablespoons

Canned and Frozen Fruits
Note: Each of the following in the amount listed is considered one Fruit Exchange (approximately 40 Calories).*

Applesauce   ½ cup water packed or artificially sweetened
⅙ cup sweetened*
Apricots   3 medium halves, water packed or artificially sweetened
2 medium halves, juice packed
1 medium half, 1 tablespoon juice, in heavy syrup*
⅙ cup frozen, sweetened*
Berry fruits other than strawberries   ½ cup packed or artificially sweetened
⅕ cup in heavy syrup*
⅔ cup frozen, unsweetened
¼ cup frozen, sweetened*
Cherries, sweet or sour   ½ cup water packed or artificially sweetened
¼ cup in heavy syrup*
½ cup frozen, unsweetened*
⅙ cup frozen, sweetened*
Figs   2 large, water packed or artificially sweetened
2 small and 1 tablespoon syrup, in heavy syrup*
Fruit cocktail   ½ cup, water packed or artificially sweetened
¼ cup in heavy syrup*
Grapefruit   ½ cup, water packed or artificially sweetened
¼ cup in heavy syrup*
Peaches   ½ cup, water packed or artificially sweetened
2 medium halves, 2 tablespoons juice, when juice packed
1 medium half, 1 tablespoon syrup, in heavy syrup*
⅕ cup, frozen, sweetened*
Pears   ½ cup, water packed or artificially sweetened
1 medium half, 1 tablespoon syrup, in heavy syrup*
Pineapple   1 large slice, water packed or artificially sweetened
1 medium slice, juice packed
½ large slice, 1 tablespoon syrup, in heavy syrup*
¼ cup, frozen, diced, sweetened*
Plums   4 medium, water packed or artificially sweetened
2 medium, 1 tablespoon syrup, in heavy syrup*
Strawberries   ¾ cup, water packed or artificially sweetened
⅕ cup, frozen, sweetened*

*Use two or more Fruit Exchanges together to give a reasonable portion.

Free Items

These may be used freely as desired.

Anchovy paste*
Bead molasses
Coffee
Condiments
Fat-free bouillon and clear broth
Herbs
Flavoring essences such as vanilla
Imitation butter flavoring
Lemon juice
Lime juice
Meat tenderizer

Meatless fat-free gravy browning
Mustard, dry or prepared
Pickled vegetables, and pickles (if sweetened, use only limited amounts)
Soy sauce
Spices
Tea
Unsweetened gelatin
Vinegar

*Use as a sauce for cooked fish or as a thin spread on crackers or in sandwiches.

Miscellaneous Exchanges and Beverages

The items in the two lists that follow, "Miscellaneous Exchanges" and "Calorie Content of Alcoholic and Carbonated Beverages," are different from those in other Exchange Groups. They provide calories, but very little in the way of essential nutrients. As used by many people, they frequently replace foods that do contain the nutrients needed by the body for proper functioning. Furthermore, these items often supply calories over and above those needed for maintaining desirable body weight. Each individual must decide for himself the quantity of these things to include in the diet, remembering that some foods are needed from each of the six groups of foods *every day*.

MISCELLANEOUS EXCHANGES

These items largely provide "empty " calories* derived from carbohydrates and are not recommended for frequent use. They may be used to fulfill a need for concentrated calorie foods after other nutritive requirements have been met. For example, in a diet of 2400 Calories or more for a man and 2000 Calories or more for a woman, one or two Fruit Exchanges may be deleted and replaced with the same number of carbohydrate exchanges, but only as indicated by the physician in the patient's individual dietary prescription.

Note: Each of the following in the amount listed is considered one Carbohydrate Exchange (approximately 40 Calories) and is equivalent in calories to one Fruit Exchange.

2 tablespoons tomato catsup
2 teaspoons honey or syrup
1 scant tablespoon jam or jelly
1 tablespoon instant cocoa

2 marshmallows
2½ teaspoons granulated sugar
2 cubes sugar
4 teaspoons powdered sugar

1 tablespoon chocolate flavored syrup
2 squares (¼ ounce) hard candy
10 small gum drops
6 jelly beans
7 (½ inch) mints

1 tablespoon packed brown sugar
3 ounces cola-type beverage
4 ounces ginger ale
3 ounces "pop"

Each amount shown may be exchanged as follows:

4 caramels—1 fat exchange and 2 bread exchanges
1 ounce sweet chocolate—2 fat exchanges and 1 bread exchange
1 ounce bitter chocolate—3 fat exchanges and ½ bread exchange
½ cup (1 scoop) sherbet—2 bread exchanges
⅓ cup Jell-O—1 bread exchange

*Calories without other significant nutritive value.

Tips on Dieting

New habits can help you both in losing weight and in keeping it off. Behavioral modification is a tremendous aid in overcoming many of the habits responsible for overeating, since excess weight has more to do with how you eat rather than what you eat. The following tips may be helpful in developing new healthy eating patterns.

- Chew your food about 15 times for each bite. You will find that your appetite is satisfied with less food.
- Never stand when eating and never eat on the run. This is a very bad habit that promotes between-meal snacking. You must sit down whenever you eat.
- After every bite, set the utensils down on your plate and pick them up again after swallowing your food. If you are eating a sandwich, a drumstick or anything you hold, also put it down after every bite.
- Do not eat unless the table is set. Set the table even when snacking.
- Always use utensils, even for popcorn, crackers or peanuts. This avoids using your fingers, thereby drastically cutting down on the amount of snacks you devour.
- Don't eat snacks while watching television. This is distracting and leads to overindulgence.
- When you are finished eating, leave the table to avoid picking.
- Make a habit of leaving something on your plate.
- Practice eating and resting intermittently at 2- to 3-minute intervals until you finish eating.
- Dole out only small servings of each item so you won't feel obliged to overeat. Moreover, if you practice more chewing and intermittent eating and resting, you will learn to satisfy your appetite with less food.
- Drink a full glass of water or begin with some bouillon or low-calorie drink just before eating to help take the edge off your hunger.

- Develop the routine of serving the salad first, and eat it slowly.
- Use smaller plates. This makes portions appear larger.
- Have meals served in the kitchen instead of placing the food at the center of the table.
- Do your food shopping after eating, never before.
- Always prepare a shopping list and stick to it.

Amount of exercise required to burn off a given number of calories.*

For example, it would take about 20 minutes of walking (at 3.5 mph) or 5 minutes of running to burn off the calories contained in an apple.

Food	Calories	Walking (3.5 mph) 5.2 calories per min.	Bike Riding 8.2 calories per min.	Swimming 11.2 calories per min.	Running 19.4 calories per min.
		Minutes of Activity			
Apple, large	101	20	12	9	5
Bacon, 2 strips	96	18	12	9	5
Banana, small	88	17	11	8	4
Beer, 1 glass	114	22	14	10	6
Bread and butter	78	15	10	7	4
Cake, 2-layer, 1/12	356	68	43	32	18
Carbonated beverage, 1 glass	106	20	13	9	5
Carrot, raw	42	8	5	4	2
Cereal, dry, 1/2 c. with milk, sugar	200	38	24	18	10
Chicken, fried 1/2 breast	232	45	28	21	12
Cookie, plain	15	3	2	1	1
Egg, fried	110	21	13	10	6
Ham, 2 slices	167	32	20	15	9
Ice Cream, 1/6 qt.	193	37	24	17	10
Malted milk shake	502	97	61	45	26
Milk, 1 glass	166	32	20	15	9
Milk, skim, 1 glass	81	16	10	7	4
Orange juice, 1 glass	120	23	15	11	6
Pancake with syrup	124	24	15	11	6
Peach, medium	46	9	6	4	2
Pie, apple, 1/6	377	73	46	34	19
Pizza, cheese, 1/8	180	35	22	16	9
Pork chop, loin	314	60	38	28	16
Club sandwich	590	113	72	53	30
Hamburger sandwich	350	67	43	31	18
Shrimp, French fried	180	35	22	16	9
Spaghetti, 1 serving	396	76	48	35	20
Steak, T-bone	235	45	29	21	12
Strawberry shortcake	400	77	49	36	21

*This chart is based on an individual weighing 150 lb.
Adapted from Konishi, F.: J. Am. Dietetic Assn. 46:186, 1965.

A service of Riker Laboratories, Inc., A Subsidiary of 3M, St. Paul, Minnesota 55144

91493

NOTE: Compiled by Riker Laboratories, Inc., from Frank Konishi, "Food Equivalents of Various Activities," *Journal of the American Dietetic Association* 46:186–188, 1965. Reprinted with permission of Riker Laboratories, Inc., and Dr. Konishi.

- Determine if any emotions are associated with your eating habits, such as anxiety, anger, tension or boredom. You may be able to modify any of these behavior patterns and substitute other avenues, such as exercise or muscle relaxation.
- Maintain a food diary and keep track of everything you eat and the circumstances during which you ate the food. Each day analyze the list with a view to correcting any "food traps" that you might circumvent or discovering any bad habits that you might correct, like taking candy snacks from the candy jar on the secretary's desk.
- Put away all visible food items, both at home and at work, and take away all serving dishes from the table. The presence of these items is a stimulus to eat. Pay heed to the wisdom of the phrase, Out of sight, out of mind.
- Take your mind off eating by developing useful hobbies such as arts, crafts, computer skills. This will keep both your hands and mind busy.

EXERCISE AND WEIGHT LOSS

Exercise alone is not a very effective means to lose weight. It takes about 26 minutes of running or 96 minutes of walking to expend about 500 calories. In terms of weight loss, you must use about 600 calories a day for one week to lose one pound. The following chart clearly shows the amount of exercise that is required to burn off the number of calories contained in various common items of food. This demonstrates that the only reliable way to lose weight is to reduce your intake of calories if you are not engaged in manual labor or are not involved in a high-level exercise program. Exercise in combination with calorie reduction is, however, very beneficial in maintaining a normal weight, in promoting cardiovascular health and in keeping the muscles firm.

Appendix D

Recipes

BASIC DAIRY PRODUCTS AND EGG SUBSTITUTES

Basic Low-Fat Milks

1. COOKING SUBSTITUTE

The following non-fat milk should be used in most recipes calling for whole milk as an ingredient.

1¼ cups non-fat dry milk solids
4 cups cold water

Mix both ingredients thoroughly, preferably with an electric mixer. Store in refrigerator.

2. BEVERAGE SUBSTITUTE

The following two recipes should be used in place of whole milk as a beverage and in coffee.

A. Low-Fat Milk

Begin by drinking 2 percent milk for three months; then go to 1 percent milk for six months, followed by skim milk. If 1 percent milk is intolerable, stay with 2 percent milk for another month; then mix one quart of 2 percent milk with one quart of 1 percent milk, which will result in 2 quarts of 1½ percent milk. Stay on this mixture for three months, then try the 1 percent milk again. Before going to skim milk, mix one quart of 1 percent milk with one quart of skim milk to make 2 quarts of ½ percent milk. You will acquire a taste for this if you have patience. So don't rush it; take your time.

B. Skim Milk, Fortified

The addition of non-fat dry milk solids is intended to provide the body with the nutrients that are lacking in skim milk. However, if calories are a problem, the milk solids need not be added.

> ½ cup non-fat dry milk solids
> 1 quart skim milk

Mix both ingredients thoroughly, preferably with an electric mixer for a light, smooth texture.

Home-made Yogurt

4 cups 2 percent milk
1½ cups water
2 heaping tablespoons commercial yogurt (when making it for the first time, but use home-made yogurt thereafter).

Place milk and water in a saucepan and heat slowly to boiling point. Remove from heat and cool until moderately warm by immersing the saucepan in cold water. Add yogurt and mix thoroughly. Cover the saucepan and set in an unheated oven until the whole mass "sets" (6 –12 hours).

Makes 5 cups
1 cup = 119 calories

Yogurt "Cream Cheese"

5 cups Homemade Yogurt (*above*)

Line a large strainer with cheesecloth and place in a bowl. Transfer the yogurt mass to the strainer and tie the ends of the cheesecloth. Put in the refrigerator and let the water drain off into the bowl for several hours.

   This recipe can be used successfully in many dishes that call for cream cheese, such as dips, spreads, and salads. Though lemon juice is usually added to most dips and spreads, it is not required for this product.

Makes about 3 cups
1 cup = 119 calories

Polyunsaturated "Sour Cream"

This recipe is an excellent substitute for the sour cream used in many recipes—for example, in dips, salads, chive dressing, and with paprika chicken and veal. (See index.)

1¼ teaspoons unflavored gelatin
⅓ cup cold water
⅓ cup boiling water
½ cup Yogurt "Cream Cheese" (*p. 192*)
¼ cup non-fat dry milk solids
¼ cup safflower or cottonseed oil

Mix gelatin with cold water until softened, then add boiling water, and stir until thoroughly dissolved. Cool until tepid. Add Yogurt "Cream Cheese" to a small electric-mixer bowl and slowly add dissolved gelatin. Mix until well blended (about 2 minutes). Freeze mixture until just stiff (about 20 minutes). Place the bowl back in the mixer, set appliance at high speed, and slowly add non-fat dry milk solids. Beat for 2–3 minutes, then slowly add polyunsaturated oil, blending thoroughly. Refrigerate mixture until ready to use.

Makes about 2½ cups
1 tablespoon serving = 17 calories

Polyunsaturated Whipped Cream Substitute

This whipped cream substitute is essentially a polyunsaturated fat with only a small percentage of saturated fats, and it is very close to the real product in both taste and consistency. It can be used whenever whipped cream is specified—for strawberry shortcake, pudding and ice cream toppings, or other desserts.

1 teaspoon gelatin
2 teaspoons cold water
3 tablespoons boiling water
½ cup ice water
½ cup non-fat dry milk solids
3 tablespoons sugar or sugar substitute to taste
3 tablespoons safflower or cottonseed oil

Mix gelatin with the 2 teaspoons of cold water until softened; then add boiling water and stir until thoroughly dissolved. Let cool until tepid. Place ice water and non-fat dry milk solids in a small, chilled electric-mixer bowl. Beat at high speed until stiff peaks form. Add sugar or sugar substitute, oil, and then gelatin. Freeze for about 15 minutes, then transfer to the refrigerator until ready to use.

Makes 1 cup

Variations:

Use chilled fruit juices instead of water.

1 tablespoon serving, if sugar used = 17 calories

1 tablespoon serving, if sugar substitute used = 15 calories

Egg Substitute

3 egg whites

2 tablespoons non-fat dry milk solids

1 teaspoon polyunsaturated oil or margarine

2 drops yellow food coloring

Mix all the ingredients in a blender or food processor. Four tablespoons of this mixture is equal to one egg.

Makes one serving

Variation: Three tablespoons of cottage cheese or tofu may be substituted for the non-fat dry milk solids.

1 serving = 146 calories

1 serving of variation = 114 calories

SPREADS AND DIPS

Polyunsaturated Spread

This spread is very easily prepared and is inexpensive. Essentially polyunsaturated-nonhydrogenated with only a small percentage of saturated fats, it should be used as a butter substitute on toast, in whipped or mashed potatoes, with lobster and vegetables, and as a base for canapé spreads (see Garlic Spread, *p. 195*; Horseradish Spread, *p. 195*). This spread cannot be used for frying because of the high content of milk solids. (If you don't have time to prepare the Polyunsaturated Spread, see pp. 180–181 for substitutes).

¾ cup ice water

¾ cup non-fat dry milk solids

3 cups polyunsaturated oil

½ teaspoon salt or salt substitute

3 drops yellow food coloring

Place ice water and non-fat dry milk solids in small, chilled electric-mixer bowl and beat at highest speed until stiff peaks form (about 5 minutes). Change to low speed and add salt or salt substitute and food coloring. Gradually add polyunsaturated oil while constantly scraping the sides of the bowl. Reduce speed. Mix just until blended. (CAUTION: Overbeating will cause the spread to become gelatinous in consistency. Let experience be your guide.) Spoon into small covered dishes and refrigerate.

Makes 4 cups
1 tablespoon serving = 95 calories

Garlic Spread
¼ cup Polyunsaturated Spread (*p. 194*) or soft, unsalted margarine
½ teaspoon garlic, minced

Blend both ingredients together. Spread on slices of French or Italian bread and toast in oven.

Makes ¼ cup
1 tablespoon serving = 24 calories

Horseradish Spread
¼ cup Polyunsaturated Spread (*p. 194*) or soft, unsalted margarine
1 tablespoon horseradish

Drain excess fluid from the horseradish through a strainer. Combine with Polyunsaturated Spread or margarine and mix until thoroughly blended.
   Excellent on small pieces of meat or on meat sandwiches.

Makes ¼ cup
1 tablespoon serving = 24 calories

Onion Dip
1 cup Polyunsaturated "Sour Cream" (*p. 193*)
1 package onion soup mix

Blend all ingredients together in an electric blender for about 2 minutes. If a blender is not available, crush onion mix, add to sour cream, and beat with a fork until well blended. Chill in refrigerator, covered, until ready to use.

Makes about 1 cup
1 tablespoon = 17 calories

Clam Dip
⅓ cup Polyunsaturated "Sour Cream" (*p. 192*) or Yogurt "Cream Cheese" (*p. 192*)
2 heaping tablespoons finely chopped onion
¼ cup minced clams
sprinkle of salt or salt substitute, to taste (optional)
1 heaping tablespoon Homemade Mayonnaise (*p. 201*) (optional)

Blend all ingredients together. Store in refrigerator.

Makes about ¾ cup
1 tablespoon = 15 calories

Garlic Dip

½ cup Polyunsaturated "Sour Cream" (*p. 193*)
1 tablespoon Roquefort cheese
¼ cup Yogurt "Cream Cheese" (*p. 192*)
½ teaspoon Worcestershire sauce
⅛ teaspoon salt or salt substitute (optional)
1 tablespoon maraschino cherry juice
¼ teaspoon garlic, minced

Blend Polyunsaturated "Sour Cream," Roquefort cheese, and Yogurt "Cream Cheese" together in an electric blender for one minute. Add Worcestershire sauce and salt or salt substitute and blend another minute. Add cherry juice and garlic and blend another minute. Chill until ready to use.

Makes about 1 cup
1 tablespoon = 14 calories

Shrimp, Crab, or Lobster Dip

1 cup finely chopped shrimp, crabmeat, or lobster
3 heaping tablespoons of Homemade Mayonnaise (*p. 201*)
1 tablespoon lemon juice
2 tablespoons finely chopped onions
½ teaspoon Worcestershire sauce
2 teaspoons maraschino cherry juice

Place shrimp, crabmeat, or lobster into a blender and add mayonnaise. Blend for about one minute; then add lemon juice and onions. Blend another minute; then add Worcestershire sauce and maraschino cherry juice and blend for 2 more minutes. Chill in refrigerator until ready to serve. If a blender is not available, chop shrimp, crabmeat, or lobster finely with a fork and mix thoroughly with mayonnaise. Add remainder of ingredients and thoroughly blend with fork.

Makes about 1½ cups
1 tablespoon Shrimp Dip = 24 calories
1 tablespoon Crab or Lobster Dip = 19 calories

SOUPS, SAUCES, AND GRAVY

Mulligatawny Soup

½ cup polyunsaturated oil
1 cup diced chicken or turkey breast
¼ cup diced onion
¼ cup diced celery
¼ cup diced carrots

2 tart apples, peeled, cored and sliced
¼ cup unbleached flour
1 teaspoon curry (or amount to taste)
6 cups chicken or turkey broth
1 cup drained canned stewed tomatoes
1 tablespoon chopped parsley
2 whole cloves
½ teaspoon salt or salt substitute (optional)

Place oil, chicken or turkey breast, onion, celery, carrots, and apples in a heavy 6-quart pot and sauté until light brown. Stir in flour and curry. Gradually add chicken or turkey broth and stir in tomatoes, parsley, cloves, and salt or salt substitute. Cover and simmer for one hour or until meat is tender. Remove cloves. Strain soup through sieve and purée the remaining solid ingredients. Stir puréed mixture back into strained broth and heat to serving temperature.

Makes 8 servings
1 serving = 188 calories.

Polyunsaturated Cream Sauce
THIN
1 tablespoon polyunsaturated oil
1 tablespoon unbleached white flour
1 cup substitute milk (*p. 191*), warmed
salt or salt substitute, to taste (optional)
sprinkle paprika
2 drops yellow food coloring
¼ teaspoon garlic, minced

MEDIUM
2 tablespoons polyunsaturated oil
2 tablespoons unbleached white flour
1 cup substitute milk (*p. 191*), warmed
salt, or salt substitute, to taste (optional)
sprinkle paprika
2 drops yellow food coloring
¼ teaspoon garlic, minced

THICK
3 tablespoons polyunsaturated oil
3 tablespoons unbleached white flour
1 cup substitute milk (*p. 191*), warmed
salt or salt substitute, to taste (optional)
sprinkle paprika
2 drops yellow food coloring
¼ teaspoon garlic, minced

Heat polyunsaturated oil in saucepan over low flame. Add flour slowly while mixing. Add warmed milk slowly, stirring constantly. Add salt or salt substitute, paprika, food coloring, and garlic. Cook in a double boiler or over very low heat, stirring constantly until mixture thickens. Cook an additional 5 minutes.

If a blender or food processor is available, add all ingredients except the milk and blend for 10 seconds; then add warmed milk slowly and blend for 10 more seconds. Pour into saucepan and proceed as above.

Makes one cup
1 tablespoon thin sauce = 15 calories
1 tablespoon medium sauce = 24 calories
1 tablespoon thick sauce = 33 calories

Lemon Polyunsaturated Spread Sauce
¼ cup Polyunsaturated Spread (*p. 194*)
3 teaspoons lemon juice
salt or salt substitute, to taste (optional)
sprinkle chopped parsley

Mix all ingredients in a double boiler and warm. Use in place of butter sauce for lobster, crab, broiled fish, and shrimp.

Makes ¼ cup
1 tablespoon = 5.6 calories

Snow Shrimp Sauce
1 cup Yogurt "Cream Cheese" (*p. 192*)
¼ teaspoon chives
salt or salt substitute, to taste
1 pound boiled shrimp, chilled
chopped lettuce

Mix cheese, chives, and salt or salt substitute. Place chilled shrimp on shredded lettuce. Serve sauce and shrimp separately.

Makes over 2¼ cups
1 tablespoon = 13 calories

Cocktail Sauce Diablo
½ cup tomato catsup
1 teaspoon prepared mustard
¼ teaspoon salt or salt substitute (optional)
1 tablespoon horseradish
1 tablespoon lemon juice
¼ teaspoon polyunsaturated oil

Combine catsup, mustard, salt or salt substitute, horseradish, lemon juice, and polyunsaturated oil in a bowl. Chill until ready to serve.

Makes about ½ cup
1 tablespoon = 10 calories

Basic Gravy
meat drippings
½–1 tablespoon polyunsaturated oil per cup of drippings
2 tablespoons unbleached white flour per cup of drippings

Remove meat drippings from roast and separate the fat by the separation technique (*p. 69*). Meanwhile, heat oil in a saucepan over low flame, add flour, and mix well. Slowly add warmed defatted meat drippings to oil and flour mixture. Stir constantly over very low heat or in double boiler until the mixture thickens. Simmer an additional 5 minutes.

If a blender or food processor is available, add oil and flour and blend 10 seconds; then slowly add hot separated drippings and blend 10 more seconds. Transfer to a saucepan and proceed as above.

Variation: Two tablespoons of black coffee may be added to beef or veal gravy for deepening the color.
1 tablespoon = 11 calories

SALADS AND DRESSINGS

Carrot Salad Supreme
6 cups carrots, shredded
2 tablespoons Homemade Mayonnaise (*p. 201*)
1 tablespoon honey
1 tablespoon polyunsaturated oil
1 tablespoon lemon juice
1 teaspoon nutmeg
½ teaspoon cinnamon
½ cup raisins

In a large bowl combine mayonnaise, honey, oil, lemon juice, nutmeg, and cinnamon. Add shredded carrots and toss thoroughly. Sprinkle with raisins and serve.

Makes 6 servings
1 serving = 146 calories

Waldorf Salad

4 cups apples, unpeeled, diced
1 cup celery, chopped
½ cup walnuts, chopped
1 tablespoon lemon juice
⅔ cup Homemade Mayonnaise (*p. 201*)

In a large bowl combine apples, celery, and nuts. Add lemon juice and mayonnaise. Toss thoroughly. Serve on lettuce leaves.

Makes 6–8 servings
1 serving = 252 calories

Cucumber Salad

2 medium-sized cucumbers, pared and sliced thin
1 small onion, chopped fine
2 scallions, chopped fine
1 small green pepper, chopped fine
salt or salt substitute, to taste (optional)
1 tablespoon lemon juice
1 cup Polyunsaturated "Sour Cream" (*p. 193*)

Place cucumbers, onion, scallions, and green pepper in salad bowl, and salt to taste. Add lemon juice and toss; then add the Polyunsaturated "Sour Cream" and toss again thoroughly. Serve chilled.

Makes 4 servings
1 serving = 107 calories

Polyunsaturated "Sour Cream" or Yogurt Salad Dressing

1 medium head of green lettuce
1 tablespoon polyunsaturated oil
2 heaping tablespoons chives, minced
1 tablespoon onion, minced
1 tablespoon lemon juice
1 cup Polyunsaturated "Sour Cream" (*p. 193*) or Homemade Yogurt (*p. 192*)
salt or salt substitute, to taste (optional)

Toss lettuce with oil, minced chives, minced onion, lemon juice, and Polyunsaturated "Sour Cream" or Homemade Yogurt. Mix thoroughly and serve chilled. This is good with cucumber and lettuce salads.

Makes 4 servings
1 serving Polyunsaturated "Sour Cream" dressing = 100 calories
1 serving Homemade Yogurt dressing = 65 calories

Low-Fat Creamy Dressing

12 ounces low-fat cottage cheese
⅛ cup low-fat milk (optional)
2 tablespoons lemon juice
2 tablespoons Homemade Mayonnaise (*p. 201*)
1 cucumber, medium size, pared and sliced

Blend all ingredients together in a blender or food processor until creamy in consistency.

Makes 4–6 servings
Variation: Dill or horseradish may be substituted for the cucumber.
1 serving = 104 calories

Low-Fat Creamy Italian Dressing

12 ounces low-fat cottage cheese
½ cup low-fat milk
1 pinch oregano
½ clove garlic, minced
2 tablespoons Homemade Mayonnaise (*p. 201*)

Blend all ingredients in an electric blender or food processor until creamy in consistency.

Makes 4–6 servings
1 serving = 107 calories

Homemade Mayonnaise

2 egg whites
2 tablespoons lemon juice or vinegar
1 teaspoon dry mustard
1 teaspoon salt or salt substitute
Egg substitute equivalent to 2 eggs (*p. 194*)
2 cups polyunsaturated oil

Place egg whites in mixing bowl or blender and beat briefly. Add one tablespoon lemon juice or vinegar, dry mustard, and salt or salt substitute. Beat briefly again. Add egg substitute; then add the oil slowly while beating at top speed. Follow with the second tablespoon of lemon juice or vinegar and beat again. The consistency of the mayonnaise depends on the amount of oil added, so add more oil slowly if a thicker mayonnaise is desired.

Makes 2½ cups
Variation: Food coloring may be added for party effects.
1 tablespoon = 102 calories

Downey Polyunsaturated Dressing
1 tablespoon Roquefort, blue, or Gorgonzola cheese
4 tablespoons boiling water
½ teaspoon garlic, minced
3 tablespoons non-fat dry milk solids
1 tablespoon onion, minced
1 tablespoon chives, minced
¼ cup lemon juice
½ cup polyunsaturated oil
1 teaspoon salt or salt substitute, to taste

Mash cheese in a bowl with the hot water. Add minced garlic, non-fat dry milk solids, onion, and chives, and mix thoroughly. In another bowl, combine lemon juice and oil; then stir into cheese mixture. Toss with salad greens until well mixed.

Makes 1¼ cups
Variation: Add about 3 tablespoons of Chianti.
1 tablespoon = 55 calories

Lemon and Oil Dressing
½ cup polyunsaturated oil
¼ cup lemon juice
¼ teaspoon garlic, minced
½ teaspoon salt or substitute (optional)
2 tablespoons minced green onion or chives
2 tablespoons non-fat dry milk solids

Blend all ingredients. Add to mixed salad greens and cucumbers and toss until thoroughly coated.

Makes about 1 cup
Variation: Add 2 or 3 tablespoons red wine, dry vermouth, or brandy.
1 tablespoon = 65 calories

Polyunsaturated "Sour Cream" Chive Dressing
1 cup Polyunsaturated "Sour Cream" (*p. 193*)
½ teaspoon lemon juice (optional)
½ teaspoon salt or salt substitute (optional)
2 tablespoons chopped chives

Mix together sour cream, lemon juice, salt or salt substitute, and chives (or blend in blender or food processor for about 10 seconds), and serve on baked potatoes or on cucumber salad or cucumber and lettuce salad.

Makes about 1 cup
Variation: Homemade Yogurt (*p. 192*) may be substituted for Polyunsaturated

"Sour Cream"
1 tablespoon = 12 calories

Russian Dressing
1 teaspoon sugar or sugar substitute
¾ cup polyunsaturated oil
¼ cup vinegar
½ cup catsup
½ teaspoon salt or salt substitute (optional)
½ teaspoon chopped parsley
pepper, to taste
1 teaspoon chives

Mix all ingredients thoroughly, place in the refrigerator for about 10 minutes, remove, mix again, and chill until ready to use. Excellent on iceberg lettuce chunks.

Makes about 1½ cups
1 tablespoon = 68 calories

Quick Chive Dressing
1 pint low-fat cottage cheese
½ cup non-fat dry milk solids
1 cup water
1 teaspoon lemon juice
1 teaspoon salt or salt substitute (optional)
2 tablespoons chopped chives
1 teaspoon onion, minced

Blend all ingredients in a blender or food processor for 20 seconds. Delicious on baked potatoes.

Makes about 3 cups
1 tablespoon = 13 calories

Cheese Horseradish Salad Dressing
2 tablespoons chives
2 tablespoons onion, finely chopped
salt or salt substitute, to taste (optional)
¼ teaspoon garlic, minced
1 tablespoon lemon juice
3 heaping tablespoons horseradish
½ cup Yogurt "Cream Cheese" (*p. 192*)

Mix all ingredients thoroughly. This dressing is delicious on lettuce and cucumber.

Makes about 1 cup
1 tablespoon = 11 calories

MEAT DISHES

Roast Veal

1 veal leg or shoulder (4–5 pounds)
1 large onion, chopped into small chunks
2 cloves garlic, slivered
1 teaspoon ginger
½ teaspoon pepper
1 tablespoon polyunsaturated oil
1½ cups water
⅛ cup lemon juice
¼ teaspoon marjoram

Preheat oven to 325 degrees.

Cut pockets in various places on the veal. Insert chunks of onion and slivers of garlic into the pockets. Season the veal all over with ginger and pepper and place on a rack in the roasting pan. Mix oil, water, lemon juice, and marjoram, and insert into various parts of the veal with an injector. (If you don't have an injector, baste veal periodically to keep moist.) Pour remainder of the mixture over the meat, cover, and bake for about 35 minutes per pound or to an internal temperature of 175 degrees.

Save the drippings for gravy.

Makes 6 servings
1 serving = 648 calories

Minted Roast Veal

1 leg of veal (about 4 pounds)
½ teaspoon dried mint leaves or 1 tablespoon fresh mint leaves
2 tablespoons polyunsaturated oil
¼ cup lemon juice
1½–2 cups of water
1 large onion, chopped
2 small garlic cloves, slivered
pepper, to taste

Preheat the oven to 325 degrees.

Blend the mint leaves with a few drops of oil and lemon juice. Then add water, remaining oil and lemon juice. Cut pockets in various places on the veal. Insert chunks of onion and slivers of garlic in the pockets. Season with pepper. Place the veal on a rack in a baking pan and baste it with the mint-leaves mixture; also insert the mixture into various parts of the veal with an injector. Cover and bake for about 35 minutes per pound or to an internal temperature of 175 degrees.

Save the drippings for gravy.

Makes 6 servings
1 serving = 602 calories

Roast Veal with Tomato Sauce

1 leg or shoulder of veal (4–5 pounds)
salt or salt substitute, to taste (optional)
pepper, to taste
1 tablespoon polyunsaturated oil
1 large onion, cut into small chunks
½ teaspoon garlic, slivered
2½ cups canned stewed tomatoes
1½ cups tomato sauce
1 teaspoon oregano
1 tomato sauce can of water

Preheat the oven to 325 degrees.
    Season veal with salt and pepper; then rub with a little oil. Cut a few small pockets in the veal and insert pieces of onion and garlic. Bake for about 35 minutes per pound or to an internal temperature of 175 degrees. Combine tomatoes, sauce oregano, and water and pour over the roast about ½ hour before it is done.

Makes 6 servings
1 serving = 746 calories

Veal Stew with Brandy

2½ pounds veal, rump or shoulder, cut into 1½-inch cubes
1 teaspoon salt or salt substitute (optional)
pepper, to taste
4 tablespoons polyunsaturated oil
2 tablespoons chives, chopped fine
1 tablespoon onions, chopped fine
⅓ cup white wine
2 tablespoons brandy
3 large fresh tomatoes or 3½ canned whole tomatoes
1¼ cups mushrooms, chopped

Season veal cubes with salt and pepper, place in a large skillet containing the polyunsaturated oil. Brown the meat on both sides; then add chives, onions, wine, and brandy. Cover and simmer for three minutes; then add tomatoes and mushrooms.
Simmer about 30 minutes or until the meat is tender.

Makes 4–6 servings
1 serving = 549 calories

Ham with Cherries

1 large canned ham, precooked (about 3 pounds)
1 tablespoon polyunsaturated oil
1 tablespoon powdered cloves

2 heaping tablespoons brown sugar
1 can (2 cups) sour, or tart, cherries with juice
¼ cup maple syrup

Preheat oven to 350 degrees.

Trim all visible fat from the ham and defat (*p. 69*). Make several deep slices about ¾" through the whole length of the ham. Rub oil over the ham and then season with cloves and brown sugar. Place the ham on a rack in a baking pan and pour sour cherries and juice between the slices. Then slowly add the maple syrup. Remove the cherry and syrup mixture from the bottom of the pan and insert some of it into various places in the meat with an injector. Set the remainder of the mixture aside for basting. Bake for about 45 minutes, basting occasionally with the mixture. Do not baste with the drippings; they should be discarded after the ham is done.

Makes 6–8 servings
1 serving = 459 calories

Baked Glazed Ham
1 canned, precooked, or fresh ham (3 pounds)
1 tablespoon ground cloves
½ cup brown sugar
1 cup applesauce

Preheat oven to 325 degrees.

Trim away all visible fat and defat (*p. 69*). Beginning at the bottom of the ham, make about 4 horizontal slices about ¾ of the way toward the top. Place ham on a rack in a baking pan. Rub well with ground cloves, then with brown sugar between the slices and over the surface. Place in oven. Carefully add the applesauce after the ham has been cooking 15 minutes, and sprinkle a little more brown sugar on top of the applesauce. The entire baking time for a precooked ham is about 40 minutes. For a fresh ham, baking time is about 20 minutes per pound or to an internal temperature of about 180 degrees. Be sure to discard the meat drippings periodically.

Makes 6–8 servings
Variations:
1. Baste with grape juice instead of applesauce.
2. Baste with orange juice instead of applesauce, and place pieces of orange in little pockets throughout the ham as well as over the top as a garnish.

1 serving = 428 calories

Broiled Chicken au Vin
1 frying chicken, cut into serving pieces (2–3 pounds)
2 tablespoons polyunsaturated oil

3 tablespoons lemon juice
2 tablespoons white wine
salt or salt substitute, to taste (optional)

Preheat oven to 350 degrees.
    Place chicken pieces in a flat pan in the broiler. Broil until brown, basting with a mixture of the oil, lemon juice, wine, and salt or salt substitute. Then transfer to preheated oven and bake for about 45 minutes or until tender.

Makes 4 servings
1 serving = 424 calories

Dutch Chicken

1 chicken fryer, cut into serving pieces (2–3 pounds)
¼ cup polyunsaturated oil
1–2 cups water
3 large stalks celery, chopped
1 large onion, chopped
⅛ teaspoon garlic, chopped
pepper, to taste

Brown chicken in a large skillet or Dutch oven with polyunsaturated oil. Add water, celery, onion, garlic, and pepper. Cover and simmer 30 to 40 minutes over a low flame

Makes 4 servings
1 serving = 498 calories

Chicken Paprika

½ cup flour
¼ teaspoon marjoram
½ teaspoon salt or salt substitute, to taste (optional)
2 teaspoons paprika
1 frying chicken, cut into serving pieces (2–3 pounds)
2 tablespoons polyunsaturated oil
1 large onion, chopped
1½ cups water
¼ teaspoon rosemary
1 tablespoon polyunsaturated oil
1 tablespoon flour
paprika
1 tablespoon lemon juice
½ cup Polyunsaturated "Sour Cream" (*p. 193*)

Place the ½ cup of flour, marjoram, salt or salt substitute, and paprika in a paper bag and shake to mix well. Heat 2 tablespoons of the polyunsaturated oil in a large skillet. Drop each piece of chicken into the paper bag, hold top closed, and shake to coat chicken thoroughly. Brown chicken on all sides in skillet. Remove chicken; then pour drippings into a bowl and reserve. Replace chicken in skillet and add onion, water, and rosemary, and simmer over low heat for about 30 minutes. Add remaining tablespoons both of polyunsaturated oil and flour. Heat slowly until liquid thickens. Add a little more paprika and 2 tablespoons of reserved drippings. Stir in lemon juice; then slowly add Polyunsaturated "Sour Cream." Simmer for 2 minutes before serving.

Makes 4 servings
1 serving = 560 calories

Old-Fashioned Meat Loaf
6 slices of day-old bread *or* 1 cup breakfast cereal (such as Cornflakes, Wheaties, Cheerios, Chex, etc.)
1 pound *very* lean ground beef or veal
1 large onion, chopped fine
3 large celery stalks, chopped fine
¼ cup parsley, chopped
1 tablespoon poultry seasoning
1 teaspoon salt or salt substitute (optional)
⅛ teaspoon pepper
2 tablespoons polyunsaturated oil
Egg substitute (*p. 194*) equivalent to 3 eggs
1 teaspoon dried mint leaves, crushed
¼ teaspoon garlic, minced
5 tablespoons unprocessed bran *or* sunflower seed kernels *or* wheat germ
1 cup tomato sauce
¼ cup water
½ teaspoon oregano

Preheat oven to 350 degrees.

In a large bowl soak the bread and press out the excess water. Add beef or veal, onion, celery, parsley, poultry seasoning, salt or salt substitute, pepper, oil, egg substitute, mint leaves, garlic; and bran, sunflower seed kernels, or wheat germ. Mix thoroughly, shape into an oval, and place in a bread pan. Cook about 30 minutes; then add tomato sauce, water, and oregano, and cook an additional 15 to 20 minutes.

Makes 6 servings
1 serving = 367 calories

SEAFOOD

Preparing a Live Lobster for Broiling

A sharp knife is required.

1. Set live lobster on its back with the claws crossed over one another. Press down firmly with the left hand.
2. Take a sharp knife and plunge into the point where the body and tail areas meet. This, which is painless, will sever the spinal cord and paralyze the lobster so that it will not move.
3. Split the lobster along the tail to the top of the head.
4. Remove the tail vein, which runs the length of the tail. Next, remove the stomach—which is located just below the head and is grayish in color—and then the lungs—the spongy organs on both sides of the cavity. If the lobster is a female, it may also contain eggs, or "coral." These eggs are considered a delicacy by gourmets.
5. The liver, or tomalley, is very tasty; it is easily identified after cooking because it turns a green color.
6. The lobster is now ready to be broiled.

Broiled Lobster with Lemon

1–1¼ lb prepared live lobster
2 tablespoons polyunsaturated oil
2 tablespoons lemon juice
¼ teaspoon paprika
salt or salt substitute, to taste (optional)
1 sprinkle of garlic (optional)

Preheat broiler.

Place lobster on a pan and brush with a mixture of the above ingredients. Broil about 4 inches from the heat for 10–15 minutes or until meat is tender. Serve with Polyunsaturated Spread (*p. 194*) or melted margarine containing a little lemon juice.

Makes one serving
Variation: Add 2 tablespoons of Chianti or white wine to the above cooking mixture.
1 serving = about 465 calories

Boiled Shrimp

1 cup water
½ teaspoon salt or salt substitute
½ stalk celery
½ teaspoon caraway seeds
1 pound shrimp

Shrimp are sold in a variety of sizes, varying from small to jumbo. It has been our experience that the smaller varieties are more succulent and less expensive than the larger. Follow these rules: (*a*) Never overboil shrimp. (*b*) Store in the stock in which they were cooked. The following technique will afford you perfectly cooked shrimp every time.

To water, add salt or salt substitute, celery, and caraway seeds, and simmer for 5 minutes. Add shrimp and cook for about 5 minutes after the water starts to boil. Serve with Diablo Sauce (*p. 198*) or Yogurt "Cream Cheese" (*p. 192*).

Makes 4 servings
1 serving = 91 calories

Broiled Fish

1½ pounds fish fillets (sole, flounder, or salmon)
sprinkle onion powder
2–3 tablespoons melted soft margarine or polyunsaturated oil
juice of 1 large fresh lemon
4–6 thin slices low-fat cheese

Preheat broiler.
Sprinkle fish thoroughly with onion powder. Squeeze lemon into melted margarine and pour half of the mixture over fish. Place cheese on top of fish and broil for 5–8 minutes. Pour the remaining margarine and lemon mix over the fish and serve.

Makes 4 servings
1 serving = 502 calories

Poached Salmon

2 pounds salmon fillet
sprinkle onion powder
1 cup dry white wine
1 cup fish or clam broth
⅛ teaspoon allspice
3 tablespoons melted soft margarine

Preheat oven to 400 degrees.
Sprinkle fish thoroughly with onion powder. Mix wine, fish or clam broth, margarine, and allspice, and pour over fish. Add additional wine, if necessary, to just cover fish. Cover with a lid or foil and bake about 15 minutes.

Makes 3–4 servings
1 serving = 345 calories

Fish Fillet in Wine Sauce

1 tablespoon polyunsaturated oil
1½–2 pounds fish fillets (sole, flounder, or salmon)
¾ cup white wine
½ teaspoon salt or salt substitute (optional)
pepper, to taste
⅛ teaspoon minced garlic (optional)
1½ tablespoons polyunsaturated oil
1½ tablespoons flour
paprika

Preheat oven to 350 degrees.

Oil a shallow baking pan. Place fillets in a large bowl. Mix white wine, salt or salt substitute, pepper, and garlic, and pour over fillets. Marinate from 15 minutes to a half hour. Place the fillets with the marinade in baking pan and bake 10–15 minutes. In the meantime, heat 1½ tablespoons of polyunsaturated oil in a skillet and add flour and paprika. Stir until a smooth paste forms; then mix in the marinade a tablespoon at a time. Heat sauce slowly until thickened, spoon over the fish, and serve.

Makes 4–6 servings
1 serving = 350 calories

Broiled Scallops

1 pound small scallops
¼ cup polyunsaturated oil
¼ teaspoon garlic, minced
½ teaspoon salt or salt substitute (optional)
⅛ teaspoon pepper
3 tablespoons lemon juice
paprika

Preheat broiler.

Dip scallops in a mixture of oil, garlic, salt or salt substitute, pepper, and lemon juice; then place on a pan and sprinkle with paprika. Broil about 4 inches from the flame for about 5 minutes or until golden brown. Be careful not to overcook; otherwise scallops will become leathery.

Makes 4 servings
Variation: Add a tablespoon of white wine to the above mixture.
1 serving = 180 calories

Baked Scallops

1 pound scallops
1 egg or egg substitute

2 teaspoons low-fat milk
pepper, to taste
⅛ teaspoon garlic, minced
5 tablespoons of polyunsaturated oil

Preheat oven to 375 degrees.

Beat the egg or egg substitute in a small bowl and add low-fat milk, pepper, and garlic. Dip the scallops into this mixture; then place in a baking pan containing the oil. Bake for about 30 minutes.

Makes 4 servings
1 serving = 220 calories

Tuna Croquettes

2 slices of bread
1½ cups canned tuna, water-packed (drained)
Egg Substitute, equivalent to one egg (*p. 194*)
1 teaspoon chopped parsley
1 teaspoon minced onion
1 teaspoon Polyunsaturated Spread (*p. 194*)
parsley sprigs for garnish

Preheat oven to 350 degrees.

In a bowl soak two slices of bread and press out excess water. Combine with tuna and blend with a fork. Mix remaining ingredients and add to tuna. Mix and shape into 6 tall cones, or croquettes. Arrange, points up, in an oiled pan and bake for about 20 minutes. During last 5 minutes of baking, add one teaspoon of Polyunsaturated Spread to the top of each croquette. Serve with a sprig of parsley.

Makes 3 servings
1 serving = 180 calories

Baked Halibut Steaks

4 medium-sized halibut steaks (about ½ pound each)
2 medium onions, sliced
4 tablespoons polyunsaturated oil
½ cup lemon juice
¼ teaspoon garlic, minced
pepper, to taste
paprika

Preheat oven to 375 degrees.

Place steaks in a baking pan that has been lightly oiled with polyunsaturated oil. Cover each of the steaks with onion slices and baste with a mixture of oil, lemon juice, garlic, and pepper. Sprinkle with paprika. Bake for about 20 minutes.

Makes 4–6 servings
Variation: Add 1 tablespoon of white wine to the basting mixture.
1 serving = 246 calories

BREAD, ROLLS, AND CEREAL

Polyunsaturated Bread

1 large (2 ounces) yeast cake
1 tablespoon sugar
1 quart warm water
3–4 tablespoons polyunsaturated oil
2 teaspoons salt or salt substitute (optional)
about 10 cups unbleached flour

In a measuring cup, crumble the yeast cake and combine with the sugar; then add ½ cup of the warm water to dissolve the yeast cake. Mix the oil, the remaining warm water, and salt or salt substitute together in a large mixing bowl. Then add the yeast mixture and mix well. Gradually sift in the flour while gently kneading, until an elastic, soft dough is formed. Place the dough in a large bowl that has been lightly greased with margarine, cover with a damp cloth, and let rise for one hour or until it has expanded to about double original size. Punch down and divide the dough into 5 loaves and place into greased bread pans. Let rise for about one hour; then bake for about 45 minutes in a preheated 350-degree oven.

Makes 5 loaves
1 slice = 56 calories

Polyunsaturated Bread Deluxe

1 large (2 ounces) yeast cake
1 tablespoon sugar
1 quart warm water
1 egg or egg substitute
3–4 tablespoons polyunsaturated oil
2 teaspoons salt or salt substitute (optional)
3–4 tablespoons honey
about 10 cups unbleached flour

In a measuring cup, crumble the yeast cake combine with the sugar; then add ½ cup of the warm water to dissolve the yeast cake. Mix egg or egg substitute, oil, the remaining warm water, salt or salt substitute, and honey together in a large bowl. Add yeast mixture and mix well. Gradually sift in flour while mixing and kneading into an elastic, soft dough. Place dough in a large bowl that has been lightly greased with margarine. Turn once. Cover lightly with a damp cloth and let rise for one hour or until about double original size. Punch down and divide dough into 5 loaves and place into greased bread pans. Let rise about one hour and bake about 45 minutes in a preheated 350-degree oven.

Makes 5 loaves
1 slice = 60 calories

Oatmeal Bread

1 large (2 ounces) yeast cake
1 tablespoon sugar
1 quart warm water
1 egg or egg substitute
3–4 tablespoons polyunsaturated oil
2 teaspoons salt or salt substitute (optional)
3–4 tablespoons honey
5 cups old-fashioned (coarse) oatmeal
about 5 cups unbleached flour

In a measuring cup, crumble the yeast cake and combine with the sugar; then add ½ cup of the warm water to dissolve the yeast cake. Mix egg or egg substitute, oil, the remaining warm water, salt or salt substitute, and honey together in a large bowl. Add yeast mixture and mix well. Stir in oatmeal. Gradually sift in flour while mixing and kneading into a soft dough. Place dough in a large bowl that has been greased with margarine. Turn once. Cover lightly with a damp cloth and let rise for one hour or until about double original size. Punch down and divide dough into 5 loaves and place into greased bread pans. Let rise about one hour; then bake about 45 minutes in preheated 350-degree oven.

Makes 5 loaves
1 slice = 52 calories

Whole Wheat Bread

1 large (2 ounces) yeast cake
1 tablespoon sugar
1 quart warm water
1 egg or egg substitute
4 tablespoons polyunsaturated oil
3 tablespoons honey
2 teaspoons salt or salt substitute (optional)
4 cups whole wheat flour
1 cup whole wheat cereal (uncooked)
about 5 cups of unbleached flour

In a measuring cup, crumble the yeast cake and combine with the sugar; then add ½ cup of the warm water to dissolve the yeast cake. Mix the egg or egg substitute, oil, the remaining warm water, honey, and salt or salt substitute in a large mixing bowl. Stir in the yeast mixture. Sift in the whole wheat flour while gently kneading. Add the whole wheat cereal; then gradually add the unbleached flour until an elastic soft dough is formed. Place the dough in a large bowl that has been lightly greased with margarine, cover with a damp cloth, and let rise for one hour or until dough has expanded to about double original size. Punch down and divide the dough into 5 loaves and place into greased bread pans. Let rise for about one hour; then bake for about 45 minutes in a preheated 350-degree oven.

Makes 5 loaves
1 slice = 57 calories

Poppy or Sesame Seed Topping for Bread or Rolls
This topping can be used on any of the bread or roll recipes in this section.
1 egg yolk
2 tablespoons low-fat milk
poppy or sesame seeds

Beat egg yolk and milk together, and brush over the top of the bread or rolls before rising. Sprinkle with poppy or sesame seeds.

Makes about 2½ tablespoons
1 tablespoon = about 28 calories

French Bread
1 regular (⅔ ounce) yeast cake
1 tablespoon sugar
2 cups warm water
1 tablespoon polyunsaturated oil
½ teaspoon salt or salt substitute (optional)
1 cup low-fat milk, warm
about 5 cups of unbleached flour

In a measuring cup, crumble the yeast cake, combine with ½ of the sugar; then add ½ cup of the warm water to dissolve the yeast cake. Mix the remaining sugar, oil, and salt or salt substitute together with the yeast mixture in a large mixing bowl and mix well. Add the remaining warm water and the warm milk, and mix. Gradually sift in the flour while gently kneading, until an elastic, soft-to-medium firm dough is formed. Place the dough in a large bowl that has been lightly greased with margarine, cover with a damp cloth, and let rise for 1–2 hours. Punch down dough and allow to rise again until it has expanded to about double original size. Punch down, knead, and divide the dough in half, forming two long loaves. Place in oiled baking pans until loaves have risen half way; then make diagonal slits across tops. Continue to let rise until double in bulk. Bake at 400 degrees for 45 minutes.

Makes 2 loaves
1 slice = 71 calories

Baking Powder Biscuits
2 cups sifted unbleached white flour
3 teaspoons baking powder

1 teaspoon sugar
½ teaspoon salt or salt substitute (optional)
3–4 tablespoons polyunsaturated oil
¾ cup low-fat milk

Sift dry ingredients together. Add the oil and blend with a fork until the dough is crumbly. Add all the milk and stir. Dough will be soft. Knead dough slightly; then roll it out on a lightly floured board into a square of about ¾″ thickness. Cut with floured biscuit cutter or small wine glass. Place on an oiled cookie sheet and bake at 400 degrees for about 15 minutes.

Makes 12 biscuits
1 biscuit = 497 calories

Bran Muffins

1 cup bran cereal
1 cup low-fat milk
1 egg or egg substitute
¼ cup honey or sugar substitute
1 tablespoon molasses
3 tablespoons polyunsaturated oil
2½ teaspoons baking powder
½ teaspoon salt or salt substitute (optional)
1 cup unbleached white flour

Preheat oven to 400 degrees.
  Combine bran and milk. Allow to stand until milk is absorbed. Mix egg or egg substitute, honey, molasses, and oil together. Add to bran mixture and mix well. Sift baking powder, salt or salt substitute, and flour together. Add to bran mixture and mix. Spoon into oiled muffin pan and bake for 25 minutes.

Makes 12 muffins
1 muffin = 120 calories

Corn Meal Muffins

1 cup corn meal
1 cup sifted unbleached flour
3 teaspoons baking powder
1 teaspoon salt or salt substitute (optional)
1 egg or egg substitute
1 cup skim milk
2 tablespoons honey
3½ tablespoons polyunsaturated oil

Preheat oven to 375 degrees.

Combine dry ingredients in a large bowl. Mix well. Blend egg or egg substitute, milk, honey, and oil together, using a blender or food processor. Pour over dry ingredients and stir until just blended. Spoon into greased muffin pan and bake for 20–25 minutes.

Makes 12 muffins
1 muffin = 145 calories

Nut Bread
2 eggs or egg substitute
2½ cups brown sugar or sugar substitute
4 cups sifted unbleached white flour
2 cups low-fat buttermilk
1¼ teaspoons baking soda
1 teaspoon baking powder
1 teaspoon salt or salt substitute (optional)
2 tablespoons polyunsaturated oil
1 cup walnuts, pecans, or other nuts, chopped

Preheat oven to 375 degrees.
Beat eggs or egg substitute and honey until creamy. Add small amounts of flour alternately with small amounts of buttermilk while continually mixing. Add baking soda, baking powder, salt or salt substitute, and oil. Blend well. Fold in nuts. Pour into 2 oiled pans and bake for 35–40 minutes.

Makes 2 loaves
1 slice = 126 calories

Homemade Granola Cereal
3 cups rolled oats
½ cup bran
½ cup wheat germ
½ cup almonds or pecans
¼ cup raisins
1 tablespoon non-fat dry milk solids
1 teaspoon cinnamon
1 cup honey
½ cup water
2 teaspoons vanilla
½ cup polyunsaturated oil

Preheat oven to 225 degrees.
In a bowl combine oats, bran, wheat germ, nuts, raisins and non-fat dry milk solids. Place the honey, water, cinnamon, and vanilla in a pan and heat gently. Add

the oil, mix, and combine with the ingredients in the bowl. Spread out on a baking sheet and bake for one hour, stirring frequently.

Makes about 7 cups
Variation: Substitute sunflower seed kernels for wheat germ, and dates for raisins. Hazelnuts and peanuts may also be used instead of the almonds or pecans.
1 cup = 546 calories

DESSERTS

Polyunsaturated Ice Cream Recipes

The following polyunsaturated ice cream recipes will delight the palate of any ice cream connoisseur. They are unique in that they are polyunsaturated-nonhydrogenated with only a small percentage of saturated fats. These products can be prepared in minutes by the homemaker with an electric mixer and readily available ingredients that can be purchased in any grocery store or supermarket. There is no ice-crystal formation or polyunsaturated oil separation. The use of safflower oil or cottonseed oil is preferred because their bland quality acts as a vehicle for the flavors. Corn oil or peanut oil leaves a definite aftertaste and should be avoided in the ice cream recipes. Sugar substitutes can be used in place of sugar in each recipe.

Each recipe makes 1½ quarts.

REMEMBER: In each ice cream recipe (1) the mixing bowl and beaters must be prechilled in the freezer, and (2) the water or fruit juices must be ice cold.

Vanilla Ice Cream
3 cups ice water
3 cups non-fat dry milk solids
1 cup sugar or sugar substitute
½ cup safflower or cottonseed oil
2 tablespoons vanilla

Place ice water and non-fat dry milk solids in a large chilled electric-mixer bowl. Beat at highest speed until stiff peaks form. Add sugar or sugar substitute and oil in a slow stream while constantly mixing. Add vanilla and blend well. Place in freezer for an hour or two until firm. Then beat again for one minute. Store in freezer.

Makes 12 servings (½ cup each)
1 serving, if sugar used = 254 calories
1 serving, if sugar substitute used = 189 calories

Lemon Ice Cream

2⅔ cups ice water
⅓ cup lemon juice (chilled)
3 cups non-fat dry milk solids
1 cup sugar or sugar substitute
¾ cup safflower or cottonseed oil
1 teaspoon lemon extract
few drops yellow food coloring

Follow directions for Vanilla Ice Cream (*p. 218*), but substitute ⅓ cup cold lemon juice for ⅓ cup water; and substitute lemon extract for vanilla. Add yellow food coloring at the end of the first beating.

Makes 12 servings (½ cup each)
1 serving, if sugar used = 254 calories
1 serving, if sugar substitute used = 231 calories

Chocolate Ice Cream

2 cups ice water
3 cups non-fat dry milk solids
1 cup chocolate syrup, chilled
1 cup sugar or sugar substitute
½ cup safflower or cottonseed oil

Place ice water, non-fat dry milk solids, and chocolate syrup in a chilled electric-mixer bowl. Beat at highest speed until stiff. Gradually add sugar or sugar substitute and oil while beating slowly. Place in freezer until ready to serve.

This recipe does not require rebeating when firm, for it does not retain as much air in the whipping process as do other ice creams.

Makes 12 servings (½ cup each)
1 serving, if sugar used = 251 calories
1 serving, if sugar substitute used = 186 calories

Strawberry Ice Cream

1 cup syrup (drained from strawberries)
2 cups ice water
3 cups non-fat dry milk solids
1 cup sugar or sugar substitute
½ cup safflower or cottonseed oil
2 cups frozen strawberries, thawed

Drain syrup from berries that are still chilled. Combine syrup, ice water, and non-fat dry milk solids in a large chilled electric-mixer bowl. Beat at highest speed until stiff peaks form. Add sugar or sugar substitute while constantly mixing; then add oil in a slow, steady stream. Blend in strawberries and place in freezer. After an hour or two, the mixture will be firm. Beat again until smooth. Store in freezer.

Makes 12 servings (½ cup each)
1 serving, if sugar used = 254 calories
1 serving, if sugar substitute used = 238 calories

Coffee Ice Cream
3 cups coffee (chilled)
3 cups non-fat dry milk solids
½ cup sugar or sugar substitute
½ cup safflower or cottonseed oil

Follow directions for Vanilla Ice Cream (*p. 218*), but substitute the chilled coffee for the ice water.

Makes 12 servings (½ cup each)
1 serving, if sugar used = 221 calories
1 serving, if sugar substitute used = 173 calories

Maple Nut Ice Cream
3 cups ice water
3 cups non-fat dry milk solids
1 cup sugar or sugar substitute
½ cup safflower or cottonseed oil
½ cup English walnuts, chopped
1 tablespoon maple extract

Follow directions for Vanilla Ice Cream (*p. 218*), but substitute maple extract for vanilla and add the nuts at the end of the first beating.

Makes 12 servings (½ cup each)
1 serving, if sugar used = 286 calories
1 serving, if sugar substitute used = 222 calories

Black Walnut Ice Cream
3 cups ice water
3 cups non-fat dry milk solids
1 cup sugar or sugar substitute
½ cup safflower or cottonseed oil
½ cup black walnuts, chopped
2 tablespoons black walnut extract

Place ice water and non-fat dry milk solids in a large chilled electric-mixer bowl and beat at highest speed until stiff peaks form. Blend in sugar or sugar substitute. Slowly add polyunsaturated oil and continue beating until well blended. Add the black walnuts and extract, blend well, and place in freezer for an hour or two. Remove from freezer and beat again until smooth. Store in freezer.

Makes 12 servings (½ cup each)
1 serving, if sugar used = 286 calories
1 serving, if sugar substitute used = 222 calories

Banana Ice Cream
3 cups ice water
3 cups non-fat dry milk solids
1 cup sugar or sugar substitute
¾ cup safflower or cottonseed oil
4–6 extra ripe bananas
1 tablespoon banana extract

Follow directions for Vanilla Ice Cream (*p. 218*), but substitute banana extract for vanilla and add bananas at the end of the first beating.

Makes 12 servings (½ cup each)
1 serving, if sugar used = 336 calories
1 serving, if sugar substitute used = 227 calories

Peach Ice Cream
1 cup syrup (drained from peaches)
2 cups ice water
3 cups non-fat dry milk solids
1 cup sugar or sugar substitute
¾ cup safflower or cottonseed oil
2 cups canned sliced peaches (chilled)

Place syrup, ice water, and non-fat dry milk solids in a large chilled, electric-mixer bowl. Beat at the highest speed until stiff peaks form. Add sugar or sugar substitute while continually beating; then add oil in a slow, steady stream. Fold in peaches and blend. Place bowl in freezer for an hour or two and then beat again until smooth. Store in freezer.

Makes 12 servings (½ cup each)
Variation: Add one teaspoon almond extract.
1 serving, if sugar used = 325 calories
1 serving, if sugar substitute used = 259 calories

Pineapple Ice Cream
2 cups ice water
3 cups non-fat dry milk solids
1 cup syrup (drained from canned or frozen pineapple)

1 cup sugar or sugar substitute
¾ cup safflower or cottonseed oil
2 cups pineapple (canned or frozen)

Place ice water, non-fat dry milk solids, and syrup in large chilled electric-mixer bowl. Beat at highest speed until stiff peaks form. Slowly add sugar while constantly mixing; then add oil in slow, steady stream until well blended. Reduce speed and blend in pineapple. Place in freezer for an hour or two until firm. Beat again at low speed until smooth. Store in freezer.

Makes 12 servings (½ cup each)
1 serving, if sugar used = 323 calories
1 serving, if sugar substitute used = 261 calories

Peppermint Ice Cream
3 cups ice water
3 cups non-fat dry milk solids
1 cup sugar or sugar substitute
¾ cup safflower or cottonseed oil
1 tablespoon peppermint extract
few drops of red food coloring

Follow direction for Vanilla Ice Cream (*p. 218*), but substitute peppermint extract for vanilla and add red food coloring at the end of the first beating.

Makes 12 servings (½ cup each)
1 serving, if sugar used = 325 calories
1 serving, if sugar substitute used = 261 calories

Orange Sherbet
1¼ cups water
1⅓ cups sugar or sugar substitute
1 tablespoon unflavored gelatin softened in ¼ cup cold water
1 tablespoon orange peel, ground
¼ cup lemon juice
2 cups orange juice
1 teaspoon safflower or cottonseed oil
1 teaspoon lemon extract
few drops of yellow and red food coloring
2 egg whites, stiffly beaten

Boil water and sugar or sugar substitute together for 5 minutes; then add gelatin, stirring constantly until it is thoroughly dissolved. Add orange peel and cool mixture to room temperature. Add lemon and orange juices, polyunsaturated oil, lemon extract, and food coloring. Blend thoroughly and place in freezer until jelling occurs. Fold into beaten egg whites and mix well. Store in freezer until ready to serve. May be garnished with chopped nuts.

Makes about 1 quart
1 serving (½ cup) = 169 calories
One ½ cup serving, if sugar used = 169 calories
One ½ cup serving, if sugar substitute used = 40 calories

Polyunsaturated Pie Crust*
2¼ cups sifted unbleached white flour
1 teaspoon salt or salt substitute (optional)
5 tablespoons low-fat milk
½ cup polyunsaturated oil

Combine flour and salt or salt substitute. In a measuring cup, mix milk and oil; then pour into dry ingredients and blend well with a fork. Shape dough into a ball and divide in two equal parts. Chill for ½ hour. Roll out one part between two sheets of waxed paper. Remove waxed paper and line an 8″ or 9″ pie pan with crust. Add filling. Cover with Flute edges and make a few slashes in top crust to release steam.

1 pie crust = 2,124 calories

This pie crust can be substituted for your own pie crust recipe and filled with any traditional filling.

Crumb Pie Crust*
16 graham crackers
¼ cup polyunsaturated oil
¼ cup honey
¼ teaspoon salt or salt substitute (optional)

Roll crackers until they are fine crumbs. Add other ingredients and blend with a fork. Press into pie pan, lining sides and bottom. Bake at 325 degrees for 10 minutes. Cool and fill. If meringue is to be used, do not prebake. The time required to brown the meringue is enough to bake the crust.

1 pie crust = 1,620 calories

See note above.

Carrot Cake
Egg substitutes equivalent to 3 eggs
1 cup honey or sugar substitute
3 cups carrots, grated
1 cup polyunsaturated oil
2 cups flour
1 teaspoon salt or salt substitute (optional)
2 teaspoons baking soda
1½ tablespoon cinnamon
1 teaspoon vanilla
1 cup pecans, chopped

Preheat oven to 350 degrees.

In mixer bowl beat egg substitutes until creamy. Add honey or sugar substitute, carrots, and oil, mixing well after each addition. In a large bowl sift together flour, salt or salt substitute, baking soda, and cinnamon. Combine with carrot mixture until just blended. Add vanilla and pecans. Pour into two greased loaf pans. Bake for 40 minutes or until an inserted toothpick comes out clean.

1 slice, if honey used = 200 calories
1 slice, if sugar substitute used = 132 calories

Poppy Seed Loaf Cake
2½ cups sifted cake flour
1 teaspoon baking soda
1 teaspoon salt or salt substitute (amount optional)
4 egg whites, beaten stiff
1 cup sugar or sugar substitute
¾ cup polyunsaturated oil
12 ounces poppy seed filling
2 tablespoons cider vinegar
1 cup minus two tablespoons low-fat milk
1 teaspoon vanilla

Preheat oven to 350 degrees.

Sift together flour, baking soda, and salt or salt substitute. Beat 4 egg whites until stiff. Place two egg yolks into mixing bowl and beat. Slowly add sugar or sugar substitute and beat again. When creamy, slowly add oil, mixing well. Add poppy seed filling and blend well. Pour vinegar into measuring cup and add low-fat milk. Add small amounts of flour mixture alternately with small amount of vinegar and milk. Add vanilla, mix well. Fold in stiffly beaten egg whites. Pour into an oiled 16″ × 4″ × 4″ loaf pan (or two regular loaf pans) which has been lined with waxed paper on the bottom. Bake for one hour. Sift confectioner's sugar over top or serve with Polyunsaturated Whipped Cream Substitute (*p. 193*).

1 slice = 120 calories

Food Analysis Tables

The following tables are included as a reference to familiarize the reader with the fat values of various food items.

The fruits and vegetables are not included because their fat content is negligible. Fish are also not included because values are conflicting. Household measures are given in addition to the amounts in grams (1 ounce equals 28.35 grams).

The data in these tables were taken from the United States Department of Agriculture, *Nutritive Value of American Foods*, Agricultural Handbook No. 456, November 1975, by Catherine F. Adams; and the United States Department of Agriculture, Home and Garden Bulletin No. 72, September 1960; the values given were obtained from foods that were in ready-to-eat form.

Fat in Grams

	Amount of food	Grams	Total	Saturated	Mono-unsaturated	Poly-unsaturated	Calories
Grain Products:							
Barley, pearly, light uncooked	1 cup	203	2.0	trace	1.0	1.0	710
*Rye bread, American, slice	1 slice	23	trace	—	—	—	55
*Pumpernickel, slice	1 slice	23	.25	—	—	—	55
Cracked wheat bread	1 slice	25	.6	.1	.2	.2	66
Whole wheat bread	1 slice	25	.8	.1	.3	.2	61
Raisin bread	1 slice	25	.7	.2	.3	.2	66
French bread, slice ½" thick	1 slice	15	.5	.1	.2	.1	66
*Italian bread, slice	1 slice	23	.7	—	—	—	62
White bread, slice	1 slice	28	.9	.2	.4	.2	76
Cake, plain, with chocolate icing, 3 × 3 × 2"	1 sector	123	17.1	6.2	7.5	2.5	453
Cake, plain, without icing, 3 × 3 × 2"	1 piece	87	11.0	5.7	3.8	0.5	315
*Cupcakes, 2¾" diam.	1 cupcake	40	3	1	2	trace	130
Pound cake, slice, 3½ × 3 × ½"	1 slice	30	8.9	2.3	4.4	1.8	142
Sponge cake, 1 cube	1 sector	66	3.8	—	—	—	196
Rolls, unenriched, rectangular	1 roll	25	.8	.2	.4	.2	78
Rolls, hard, 12–22 oz.	1 roll	50	1.6	.4	.7	.4	156
Spaghetti with meat sauce	1 cup	248	11.7	3.3	6.3	.9	332
Nuts, Peanuts, and Related Products:							
*Almonds, shelled	1 cup	142	77	6	52	15	850

*Brazil nuts, broken pieces	1 cup	140	92	18	44	24	905
Cashew nuts, roasted	1 cup	140	64.0	10.9	44.8	4.5	785
Coconut, fresh, shredded	1 cup	80	28.2	24.3	2	trace	277
Peanuts halves, roasted, shelled	1 cup	144	70.1	15.4	30.2	20.3	838
Peanuts, chopped, roasted	1 tablespoon	9	4.4	1.0	1.9	1.3	52
Peanut butter	1 tablespoon	16	8.1	1.5	3.8	2.3	90
*Pecans, halves	1 cup	108	77	5	49	15	740
*Pecans, chopped	1 tablespoon	7.5	5	trace	3	1	50
*Walnuts, shelled, black, chopped	1 cup	126	75	4	26	36	790
*Walnuts, English or Persian, halves	1 cup	100	64	4	10	40	650
*Walnuts, English or Persian, chopped	1 tablespoon	8	5	trace	1	3	50
Eggs:							
Raw (whole without shell) med.	1 egg	50.0	5.1	1.6	2.2	.4	72.0
White of egg	1 white	35.0	trace	.1	.2	.1	15.0
Yolk of egg	1 yolk	15.0	4.6	1.5	2.0	.3	52.0
Meats, Poultry, Fish and Shellfish:							
Bacon	2 slices	15.0	7.8	2.5	3.7	.7	86.0
*Beef (lean and fat)	3 oz.	85.0	16.0	8.0	7.0	trace	245.0
Hamburger, broiled, market ground	3 oz.	85	9.6	4.6	4.2	.2	186

*Designates values from United States Department of Agriculture Home and Garden Bulletin No. 72, September 1960.

Fat in Grams (continued)

Amount of food	Grams	Total	Saturated	Mono-unsaturated	Poly-unsaturated	Calories
*Ground lean	3 oz.	85	10.0	5.0	4.0	trace	185
Beef, canned, corned beef	1 slice	40	4.8	2.3	2.1	.1	86
Corned beef hash	1 cup	220	24.9	11.9	10.9	.5	398
*Beef, dried or chipped	2 oz.	57	4.0	2.0	2.0	trace	115
*Chicken (flesh and skin only) (½ breast fried)	2.8 oz.	79	12.0	3.0	6.0	2	215
*Chicken, leg, fried (trimmed of fat)	3.1 oz.	89	15.0	4.0	7.0	2	245
Lamb chop (lean and fat) broiled	4 oz.	95	27.9	15.6	10.0	.8	362
Leg, lamb (roasted)	8 oz.	227	42.8	24.4	15.4	1.3	633
Shoulder, lamb (lean and fat), roasted	9½ oz.	270	73.5	41.1	26.4	2.2	913
Liver, beef, fried	1 slice	85	9.8	2.9	3.8	1.4	195
Pork, ham, baked or roasted	4.1 oz.	131	40.1	14.4	16.8	3.6	490
Bacon, medium	2 slices	15	7.8	2.5	3.7	.7	86
Bologna	1 oz. (1 slice)	28	6.5	—	—	—	79
Cooked ham, luncheon meat	1 oz. (1 slice)	28	4.8	1.7	2.0	.4	66
Canned, pork, luncheon meat, (spiced or unspiced)	1 oz. (1 slice)	28	7.0	2.5	3.0	.5	82
Pork chop, broiled	2 oz.	58	18.4	—	—	—	227
Pork roast (lean and fat) 84% lean—16% fat	6.5 oz.	186	41.1	14.8	17.2	3.7	490
Frankfurter, cooked	1 frankfurter	45	12.4	—	—	—	139

Tongue, beef, simmered	1 slice	20	3.3	1.6	1.4	trace	49
Veal cutlet, broiled	3 oz.	85	9.0	4.0	4.0	trace	185
Veal roast, medium done (lean and fat)	3 oz.	85	9.4	4.5	4.1	.2	184
Bluefish, baked or broiled	3 oz.	85	4.5	—	—	—	135
*Clams, raw meat only	3 oz.	85	1.0	—	—	—	70
*Crabmeat, canned or cooked	3 oz.	85	2.0	—	—	—	90
*Fish sticks, breaded, cooked, frozen; stick, 3.8 × 0.5″	8 oz. pack	227	20	5.0	4.0	10	400
*Haddock, fried	3 oz.	85	5.0	1.0	3.0	trace	135
Mackerel	1 oz.	28	4.5	—	—	—	67
Oysters (raw), 13–19 med. selects	1 cup	240	4.0	—	—	—	160
*Salmon, pink, canned	4 oz.	138	15.8	4.8	4.6	2.5	238
*Sardines, canned in oil	3 oz.	85	9.0	2.0	2	4.0	180
*Shrimp, canned, meat only	3 oz.	85	1.0	—	—	—	110
*Swordfish, broiled with butter	3 oz.	85	5.0	—	—	—	150
Halibut	1 oz.	28	2.0	—	—	—	
Tuna, solid pack in soybean oil	7 oz.	198	40.6	7.5	8.2	17.2	570
Milk, Cow's: Fluid, whole	1 cup	244	8.5	4.7	2.8	.2	159.0
Lowfat with 2% added milk solids	1 cup	246	4.9	2.7	1.6	.1	

*Designates values from United States Department of Agriculture Home and Garden Bulletin No. 72, September 1960.

Fat in Grams (continued)

Amount of food	Grams	Total	Saturated	Mono-unsaturated	Poly-unsaturated	Calories
Buttermilk	1 cup	246	trace	—	—	—	90.0
Evaporated, canned	1 cup	252	19.9	10.9	6.6	.6	345.0
Condensed	1 cup	306	26.6	14.7	8.8	.8	982.0
*Dry (nonfat)	1 cup	80	1.0	—	—	—	290
Skim milk	1 cup	245	.2	—	—	—	88.0
Yogurt (partially skimmed) milk	1 cup	245.0	4.2	2.3	1.4	.1	123.0
Cream:						
Half and half	1 cup	242	28.3	15.6	9.3	.8	324.0
Light (20.6% fat)	1 cup	240	49.4	27.2	16.3	1.5	506.0
*Medium	1 cup	239	78.0	43.0	26.0	2.0	745.0
*Medium	1 tablespoon	15	6.0	3.0	2.0	trace	45.0
Heavy (37.6% fat)	1 cup	238	89.5	49.2	29.5	2.7	838.0
*Heavy	1 tablespoon	15	6.0	3.0	2.0	trace	55.0
Cheese:						
Blue mold	1 ounce	28.0	8.6	4.8	2.9	.3	104.0
Cheddar (domestic) sliced	1 slice	24.0	7.7	4.3	2.6	.2	96.0
Cottage (creamed) 4.2% milk fat	1 cup	225.0	9.5	5.2	3.1	.3	239.0
*Cottage (uncreamed)	1 cup	225.0	1.0	trace	trace	trace	195.0
Creamed cheese	1 oz.	28.0	10.7	5.9	3.5	.3	106.0
Swiss (domestic)	1 oz.	28.0	7.9	4.4	2.6	.2	105.0

Milk Desserts:

Ice cream (⅛ of qt. brick) 10% fat	1 slice	66.0	7.0	3.8	2.3	.2	127.0
Ice milk (⅛ of qt. brick) 5% fat	1 slice	65.5	3.35	1.85	1.1	.1	99.5

Fats and Oils:

Butter, 4 sticks/lb., 2 sticks	1 cup	227.0	183.9	101.1	60.7	5.5	1625.0
Butter, ⅛ stick	1 tablespoon	14.2	11.5	6.3	3.8	.3	102.0
Fats, cooking lard	1 cup	205.0	205.0	77.9	94.3	20.5	1849.0
*Vegetable fats, cooking	1 cup	200.0	200.0	46.0	130.0	14.0	1770.0
Margarine, 4 sticks/lb., 2 sticks	1 cup	227.0	183.9	33.6	94.1	50.3	1684.0
Margarine, ⅛ stick	1 tablespoon	14.2	11.5	2.1	5.9	3.1	102.0
Mayonnaise, salad dressing	1 tablespoon	14.0	11.2	2.0	2.4	5.6	101.0

Sweets:

*Caramels, candy	1 oz.	28.0	3.0	2.0	1.0	trace	120.0
Chocolate, sweetened milk	1 oz.	28.6	9.2	5.1	3.3	.2	147.0
Chocolate, bitter or unsweetened	1 oz.	28.0	15.0	8.4	5.6	.3	143.0
Chocolate, sweetened	1 oz.	28.0	10.0	5.6	3.7	.2	150.0

Miscellaneous:

Cream soup (asparagus, celery)	1 cup	245.0	10.3	1.8	3.0	4.6	176.0

*Designates values from United States Department of Agriculture Home and Garden Bulletin No. 72, September 1960.

Fats in Common Foods

	Amount of food analyzed		Total fats	Percentage of fats	
		IN GRAMS	IN GRAMS	POLY-UNSAT-URATED	SAT-URATED
FATS IN COMMON DAIRY PRODUCTS					
Cheese:					
Blue mold	1 oz.	28	9	3.5	55.8
Cream cheese	1 oz.	28	11	2.8	55.0
Cheddar (ungrated)	1″ cube	17	6	2.6	55.8
Cottage (creamed)	1 cup	225	11	3.2	54.7
Swiss	1 oz.	28	8	2.5	55.7
Uncreamed cottage	1 cup	225	1	trace	trace
Cream:					
Half and half	1 cup	242	29	2.8	55.1
Heavy	1 cup	238	93	3.0	55.0
Light	1 cup	240	52	3.0	55.0
*Medium	1 cup	239	78	2.6	55.1
Milk:					
Buttermilk	1 cup	246	trace	trace	trace
Condensed	1 cup	306	25	3.0	55.2
Evaporated	1 cup	252	20	3.0	54.8
Whole milk	1 cup	244	10	2.4	55.2
Yogurt	1 cup	245	4	2.4	54.7
Skim milk	1 cup	245	.2	—	—
Dry (nonfat)	1 cup	80	1	—	—
Milk Desserts:					
Ice cream	1 slice	71	9	2.9	54.2
Ice milk	1 cup	187	10	3.0	55.2
FATS IN COMMON MEATS AND POULTRY					
Bacon	2 slices	15	7.8	9.0	32.05
Beef (lean and fat)	3 oz.	85	16	trace	50
*Beef, dried or chipped	2 oz.	57	4	trace	50
*Beef, ground lean	3 oz.	85	10	trace	50
*Beef liver	2 oz.	57	4	trace	50
*Beef, market ground	3 oz.	85	17	trace	47
Corned beef	3 oz.	85	10	2.0	47.9

*Designates values from United States Department of Agriculture Home and Garden Bulletin No. 72, September 1960.

Fats in Common Foods (continued)

	Amount of food analyzed		Total fats	Percentage of fats	
		IN GRAMS	IN GRAMS	POLY-UNSAT-URATED	SAT-URATED
Corned beef hash	3 oz.	85	5	2.0	47.8
Lamb chop (lean and fat)	4 oz.	112	33	2.9	55.9
Lamb, leg, roasted	3 oz.	85	16	3.0	57.0
Lamb shoulder, roasted	3 oz.	85	23	3.0	55.9
Pork, ham, smoked	3 oz.	85	24	8.8	35.9
Frankfurter, cooked	1 oz.	51	14	7.1	42.9
Chicken:					
*Breast, fried, ½ breast	2.8 oz.	79	12	16.7	25.0
*Leg, fried (thigh and drumstick)	3.1 oz.	89	15	13.6	26.7

FATS IN COMMON NUTS

Almonds, shelled	1 cup	142	77	19.4	7.9
Brazil nuts	1 cup	140	92	26.1	19.6
Cashew nuts	1 cup	135	65	7.0	17.0
Coconut, fresh	1 cup	97	31	trace	86.2
Peanuts, halves	1 cup	144	71	29.0	22.0
Pecans, halves	1 cup	108	65	19.4	6.49
Walnuts, black, chopped	1 cup	126	75	48	5.3
Walnuts, English, halves	1 cup	100	64	74.0	4

*Designates values from United States Department of Agriculture Home and Garden Bulletin No. 72, September 1960.

Comparison of Fats

(given in grams of fat per ounce of oil)

OIL	Food Amount HOUSEHOLD	GRAMS	CALORIES	TOTAL FATS GMS/OUNCE	TOTAL SATURATED GMS/OUNCE	MONOUN-SATURATED (LINOLEIC) GMS/OUNCE	POLYUN-SATURATED (LINOLEIC) GMS/OUNCE	APPROXIMATE # OF TBS. OF OIL TO PROVIDE 1 OZ. OF POLYUN-SATURATES
Safflower	tablespoon	13.6	120	27.25	2.18 (8%)	4.08 (15.0%)	19.61 (71.9%)	2.8
Corn	tablespoon	13.6	120	27.25	2.72 (10%)	7.63 (28%)	14.44 (53.0%)	3.8
Soybean	tablespoon	13.6	120	27.25	4.08 (15%)	5.45 (20%)	14.16 (52%)	3.8
Cottonseed	tablespoon	13.6	120	27.25	6.81 (25%)	5.72 (21%)	13.62 (50%)	4.0
Sesame	tablespoon	13.6	120	27.25	3.82 (14%)	10.35 (38%)	11.44 (42%)	4.8
Peanut	tablespoon	13.5	119	27.00	4.86 (18%)	12.69 (47%)	7.83 (29%)	7.0
Olive	tablespoon	13.5	119	27.00	2.97 (11%)	20.52 (76%)	1.89 (7%)	28.6

Cholesterol, Fat, and Fatty Acid Content of Various Foodstuffs

	Cholesterol (MG/100 GM FOOD)	Fat (GM/100 GM FOOD)	Saturated Fat (GM/100 GM FOOD)
Fish			
White fish, clams, scallops, oysters, and water-packed tuna	66	0.9	0.2
Shrimp, crab, lobster	112	1.7	0.2
Salmon	75	6.9	1.7
Poultry			
Chicken and turkey, no skin	87	1.9	1.3
Duck and goose, skin	91	33.4	8.0
Veal			
10 percent fat-trimmed roasts and chops, veal cutlets	99	11.1	4.7
15 percent fat-untrimmed loin roasts and chops	99	16.9	7.1
Beef, Pork, and Lamb			
10 percent fat-ground sirloin, trimmed lean beef and lamb	90	10.0	3.7
15 percent fat-ground round, untrimmed lean beef, trimmed lean pork	90	14.8	5.5
20 percent fat-ground chuck, untrimmed beef and lamb roasts, trimmed fatter beef and lamb	90	19.1	8.3
30 percent fat-ground beef and pork, shortribs, untrimmed, well-marbled steaks, chops (T-bone, etc.), ham	90	30.7	12.9
40 percent fat-spareribs, country-style ribs	90	38.9	10.5
Organ Meats	300–2000	4.8	1.6
Eggs			
White	0	0	0
Egg substitutes	0	4.2	1.2
Whole	504	11.5	3.4

NOTE: Reprinted with permission from O'Connor, W. E., and O'Connor, S. L., "The Dietary Treatment of Hyperlipidemia," in *The Medical Clinics of North America* 66: 485–518, 1982.

Cholesterol, Fat, and Fatty Acid Content of Various Foodstuffs (continued)

	Cholesterol (MG/100 GM FOOD)	Fat (GM/100 GM FOOD)	Saturated Fat (GM/100 GM FOOD)
Visible Fats:			
Most vegetable oils	0	100.0	13.0
Soft vegetable margarines	0	81.0	16.0
Soft shortenings	0	100.0	25.8
Butter	227	81.0	49.8
Coconut oil, palm oil, cocoa butter (chocolate)	0	100.0	74.6
Cheeses:			
Count-Down, dry-curd cottage cheese, tofu (bean curd), pot cheese, low-fat cottage cheese, St. Otho	6	2.1	0.9
Cottage cheese, Lite-Line, Chef's Delight, Breeze, Light n' Lively, part-skim ricotta	29	7.5	4.6
Cheezola, Scandic or Min Chol Hickory Farm Lyte, Pizza Pal, Saffola American*	12	24.5	4.7
Green River (lower-fat cheddar), part-skim mozzarella, Neufchatel (lower-fat cream cheese), Keil Kase, Skim American	58	18.2	10.2
Cheddar, Roquefort, Swiss, Brie, jack, American, cream cheese, Velveeta, cheese spreads (jars)	106	35.0	20.6
Frozen Desserts:			
Water ices	0	0	0
Sherbet or frozen yogurt	4	1.2	0.8
Ice milk	14	5.1	3.2
Ice cream, 10 percent fat	40	10.6	6.6
Milk:			
Skim milk (0.1 percent fat) or buttermilk	2	0.1	0.1

*Cheeses made with skim milk and vegetable oils.

Cholesterol, Fat, and Fatty Acid Content of
Various Foodstuffs (continued)

	Cholesterol (MG/100 GM FOOD)	Fat (GM/100 GM FOOD)	Saturated Fat (GM/100 GM FOOD)
1 percent milk	3	1.0	0.6
2 percent milk	6	2.0	1.2
Whole milk (3.5 percent fat)	14	3.5	2.2
Liquid non-dairy creamers: store brands, Cereal Blend, Coffee Rich	0	11.0	8.5
Liquid non-dairy creamers: Mocha Mix, Poly Rich, Mello	0	9.8	2.7

ADDENDUM BY THE AUTHOR

Cholesterol, Fat, and Fatty Acid Content of
Various Foodstuffs

	Cholesterol (MG/100 GM FOOD)	Fat (GM/100 GM FOOD)	Saturated Fat (GM/100 GM FOOD)	Calories Per Tablespoon
Margarines:				
Mazola, unsalted	0	78.6	14.3	100.0
Fleischmann's, unsalted	0	78.6	14.3	100.0
Chiffon, soft	0	76.9	15.3	90.0
Weight Watchers, unsalted	0	42.9	6.0	50.0
Diet Mazola	0	42.9	6.0	50.0
Fleischmann's Light Corn Spread	0	57.1	14.3	80.0

Dietary Fiber and Carbohydrate Composition of Common Foods

All values are given as grams per 100 grams, except for cholesterol, which is given in milligrams. *Italic* type indicates cooked foods.

Food	PROTEIN	Carbohydrate			FAT	CHOL (mg)	Fiber			CAL
		TOTAL	COMPLEX	SIMPLE			TOTAL	CRUDE	SOLUBLE	
Milk products										
Skim milk	3.4	4.9	0	4.9	0.2	1.6	—	—	—	35
powdered skim milk	35.0	52.2	0	52.2	0.7	18.7	—	—	—	358
evaporated skim milk	7.5	11.3	0	11.3	0.2	3.9	—	—	—	78
skim milk yogurt	5.7	7.7	0	7.7	0.2	1.8	—	—	—	56
1% milk	3.3	4.8	0	4.8	1.1	4.1	—	—	—	42
2% milk	3.3	4.8	0	4.8	1.9	7.4	—	—	—	50
2% yogurt	5.3	7.0	0	7.0	1.6	6.2	—	—	—	63
whole milk*	3.3	4.7	0	4.7	3.4	13.5	—	—	—	62
condensed milk*	6.8	10.0	0	10.0	7.6	29.4	—	—	—	134
yogurt, whole milk*	3.5	4.7	0	4.7	3.2	12.8	—	—	—	62
A vegetables										
beans, green	1.5	2.6	1.4	1.2	0.1	—	2.3	1.5	0.8	17
bean sprouts, mung	3.8	4.6	2.4	2.2	0.2	—	1.8	1.2	0.6	34
broccoli	3.1	2.4	1.0	1.4	0.2	—	3.2	1.1	2.1	19
cabbage	1.1	2.7	0	2.7	0.2	—	2.2	0.8	1.4	15
cabbage	1.3	3.4	0	3.4	0.2	—	2.8	1.1	1.7	19
carrots	0.8	4.0	0.1	3.9	0.1	—	2.1	0.7	1.4	19
cauliflower	1.9	2.3	0.2	2.1	0.2	—	1.2	0.9	0.3	16
celery	0.8	1.0	0	1.0	0.1	—	2.4	1.8	0.6	7
celery	0.9	1.3	0.1	1.2	0.1	—	3.0	2.2	0.8	9
cucumbers	0.8	2.6	0	2.6	0.1	—	1.5	0.4	0.9	14
green pepers	1.2	3.6	1.6	2.0	0.2	—	1.2	1.2	0	20
lettuce	1.2	1.0	0.2	0.8	0.2	—	1.5	0.9	0.6	9

mushrooms	2.7	1.9	1.8	0.1	0.3	—	2.5	1.6	0.9	17
spinach	3.2	0.8	0.1	0.7	0.3	—	3.5	2.1	1.4	14
summer squash	0.9	1.6	0.3	1.3	0.1	—	2.2	1.2	1.0	9
summer squash	1.1	2.1	0	1.7	0.1	—	3.0	1.6	1.4	12
tomatoes	1.0	3.1	0	3.1	0.2	—	1.3	1.0	0.3	18
tomatoes	1.1	3.4	0	3.4	0.2	—	1.4	1.0	0.4	19
zucchini	1.2	1.8	0.2	1.6	0.1	—	3.0	2.6	1.4	11
B vegetables										
asparagus	2.5	3.3	1.0	2.3	0.2	—	1.7	1.2	0.5	22
asparagus	2.6	3.9	2.2	1.7	0.3	—	1.3	0.9	0.4	25
beets	1.0	6.7	1.0	5.7	0.1	—	2.1	1.2	0.9	30
brussels sprouts	3.2	4.2	1.6	2.6	0.2	—	2.1	1.2	0.9	28
carrots	1.1	6.8	0.2	6.6	0.2	—	3.7	1.2	2.5	32
cauliflower	2.7	3.5	0.4	3.1	0.2	—	1.8	1.3	0.5	23
eggplant	1.2	4.1	0.3	3.8	0.2	—	1.5	0.4	0.9	22
kale	3.0	2.7	0.5	2.2	0.5	—	2.0	1.2	0.8	23
onions	1.5	6.7	1.3	5.4	0.1	—	2.1	1.1	1.0	32
onions	1.2	5.0	1.0	4.0	0.1	—	1.6	0.8	0.8	24
peas	4.8	8.0	3.4	4.6	0.4	—	6.4	4.0	2.4	53
radishes	1.0	3.1	0	3.1	0.1	—	2.2	1.7	0.5	16
turnips	1.0	4.4	1.3	3.1	0.2	—	2.2	1.2	1.0	22
C vegetables										
corn	2.5	13.8	13.1	0.7	0.7	—	3.8	2.7	1.1	72
parsnips	1.7	12.7	8.5	4.2	0.5	—	4.9	4.4	0.5	60

*not recommended but included for comparison purposes

NOTE: Reprinted from "For Diabetes, A Return to Innocence" in *Emergency Medicine*, Sept. 15, 1979, with permission of James W. Anderson, M.D.

Dietary Fiber and Carbohydrate Composition of Common Foods (continued)

Food	PROTEIN	Carbohydrate TOTAL	COMPLEX	SIMPLE	FAT	CHOL (mg)	Fiber TOTAL	CRUDE	SOLUBLE	CAL
potatoes, sweet	1.7	21.9	17.6	4.3	0.4	—	4.0	1.8	2.2	100
potatoes, white	2.1	15.7	15.0	0.7	0.1	—	3.5	1.5	2.0	73
spaghetti, macaroni	4.5	26.6	25.0	0.8	0.4	—	0.5	0.5	0.1	133
rice, brown	2.5	23.7	23.0	0.7	0.6	—	1.8	1.8	0	113
rice, white	2.0	23.6	23.1	0.7	0.1	—	0.6	0.6	0	108
barley, dry	8.2	67.7	62.0	5.7	1.0	—	11.1	10.7	0.4	322
squash, winter	1.1	6.9	3.9	3.0	0.3	—	2.9	2.6	0.3	34
kidney beans	7.8	16.6	13.6	3.0	0.5	—	4.8	4.3	0.5	101
lima beans	20.4	60.3	56.8	3.5	1.6	—	3.7	3.3	0.4	337
white beans	7.8	16.5	13.2	3.0	0.6	—	4.7	4.2	0.5	101
pinto beans	22.9	53.7	47.7	6.0	1.8	—	10.0	9.0	1.0	320
Fruit										
applesauce, unsweetened	0.2	7.7	0.5	7.2	0.2	—	1.4	0.6	0.8	35
apple	0.2	10.4	0.6	9.8	0.6	—	3.4	1.4	2.0	48
apricots, canned	0.7	8.5	0.5	8.0	0.1	—	1.3	0.5	0.8	38
apricots	1.0	11.5	0.7	10.8	0.2	—	1.7	0.7	1.0	51
banana	1.1	20.1	5.1	15.0	0.2	—	1.8	0.9	0.9	86
blackberries	1.2	7.4	1.1	6.3	0.9	—	5.0	4.1	0.9	41
strawberries	0.7	6.3	0.6	5.7	0.5	—	2.1	1.3	0.8	32
cherries	1.3	12.7	0.2	12.5	0.4	—	1.2	0.8	0.4	58
grapes	0.6	16.1	0	16.1	0.3	—	0.8	0.6	0.2	67
grapefruit	0.5	9.8	0.4	9.4	0.1	—	1.3	0.4	0.9	42
muskmelon	0.7	7.5	0	7.5	0.1	—	1.2	0.9	0.3	33
peaches, canned	1.0	10.0	0.4	9.6	0.2	—	2.1	0.5	1.6	45
orange	0.4	8.5	0.6	7.9	0.1	—	1.1	0.5	0.6	36

peach	0.6	10.4	0.7	9.7	0.1	—	1.3	0.6	0.7	44
pears, canned	0.2	8.2	1.2	7.0	0.1	—	1.3	1.0	0.3	33
pear	0.7	15.5	2.2	13.3	0.4	—	2.4	1.8	0.6	67
pineapple	0.4	12.2	0.6	11.6	0.2	—	1.0	0.7	0.3	52
plum	0.5	10.4	0.5	9.9	0.2	—	1.8	0.8	1.0	45
tangerine	0.8	9.0	0	9.0	0.2	—	2.1	0.5	1.6	40
apple juice	0.1	11.9	0	11.9	0	—	0.1	0	0.1	47
cranberry juice	0.1	16.5	0	16.5	0.1	—	0	0	0	66
grape juice	0.2	16.6	0	16.6	0	—	0	0	0	66
lemon juice	2.3	37.4	0	37.4	0.9	—	0	0	0	116
orange juice	0.8	11.0	0	11.0	0.2	—	0.3	0	0.3	48
Cereals										
rolled oats	14.2	57.0	56.4	0.6	7.4	—	9.0	6.0	3.0	350
grits	8.7	69.4	63.9	5.5	0.8	—	10.6	7.3	3.3	320
cracked wheat	10.4	61.7	51.4	10.3	2.1	—	11.1	10.7	0.4	296
All-Bran	12.6	40.8	22.3	8.5	3.0	—	33.1	33.1	0	219
shredded wheat	9.9	67.7	66.4	1.3	2.0	—	12.2	11.8	0.4	337
Grape-Nuts	11.7	65.1	63.8	1.3	3.0	—	11.2	11.0	0.2	319
Bran Buds	10.2	48.9	25.9	23.0	3.0	—	29.7	29.8	0.9	250
wheat flakes	10.2	67.4	56.2	11.2	1.6	—	13.1	12.7	0.4	333
cornflakes	7.9	72.1	66.4	5.7	0.4	—	11.0	7.6	3.4	334
farina	11.4	71.8	69.7	2.1	1.5	—	3.1	3.0	0.1	360
oat bran	22.1	45.1	44.6	0.5	6.9	—	27.6	18.4	9.2	329
Breads										
rye flour	9.1	42.2	41.0	1.2	1.2	—	10.8	10.5	0.3	214
whole wheat bread	9.1	40.4	39.2	1.2	2.6	—	9.5	9.2	0.3	224
graham crackers, plain	8.0	63.2	61.3	1.9	9.4	—	10.1	9.8	0.3	373

*not recommended but included for comparison purposes

Dietary Fiber and Carbohydrate Composition of Common Foods (continued)

Food	PROTEIN	Carbohydrate			FAT	CHOL (mg)	Fiber			CAL
		TOTAL	COMPLEX	SIMPLE			TOTAL	CRUDE	SOLUBLE	
rye crackers	13.0	65.8	65.8	2.0	1.2	—	11.7	11.4	0.3	326
flour, whole wheat	13.3	59.6	57.8	1.8	2.5	—	9.5	9.2	0.3	319
HCF whole wheat muffin	8.0	31.2	26.7	4.5	3.2	—	6.5	6.4	0.1	187
HCF corn muffin	6.6	38.8	35.1	3.7	0.7	—	3.6	2.7	0.9	194
rye flour, dark	16.3	54.2	52.6	1.6	2.6	—	13.9	13.5	0.4	298
corn bread	7.4	25.6	24.3	1.3	7.2	—	3.4	2.3	1.1	193
French bread	9.1	52.4	50.9	1.5	3.0	—	2.9	2.8	0.1	282
white bread	8.7	47.5	46.1	1.4	3.2	—	2.7	2.6	0.1	265
saltine crackers	9.0	57.9	56.2	1.7	12.0	—	3.9	3.8	0.1	380
white flour	10.5	72.9	70.1	2.1	1.4	—	3.2	3.1	0.1	360
Meat exchanges										
beef, lean	32.0	0	0	0	8.3	65	—	—	—	211
pork, ham	25.6	0	0	0	8.8	60	—	—	—	189
pork roast	25.9	0	0	0	13.0	88	—	—	—	228
chicken, light meat	31.5	0	0	0	4.3	79	—	—	—	173
turkey, light meat	32.8	0	0	0	2.6	77	—	—	—	163
cod	16.5	0	0	0	0.7	50	—	—	—	77
flounder	14.9	0	0	0	1.2	60	—	—	—	75
trout	19.2	0	0	0	4.5	60	—	—	—	123
tuna	29.0	0	0	0	6.8	60	—	—	—	185
1% cottage cheese	12.4	2.7	0	2.7	1.0	9	—	—	—	72
cheese, countdown	24.0	10.0	0	10.0	1.0	5	—	—	—	150
egg whites	10.9	0.8	0	0.8	0	0	—	—	—	51
ground beef	18.2	0	0	0	29.3	95	—	—	—	342
steak, lean	26.8	0	0	0	16.2	125	—	—	—	261

veal, loin	22.7	0	0	0	15.3	90	—	—	—	234
breakfast patty (sausage substitute)	17.2	6.6	6.6	1.3	18.5	107	—	—	—	242
cheddar cheese	25.2	1.3	0	1.6	33.6	96	—	—	—	408
American cheese	22.4	1.6	0	1.6	31.6	96	—	—	—	380
cottage cheese	12.5	2.7	0	2.7	4.5	19	—	—	—	103
eggs	12.8	0.7	0	0.7	11.5	550	—	—	—	162
egg substitute	11.0	3.0	0	3.0	12.4	0	—	—	—	171
Fatty foods										
margarine, bar	0.6	0.4	0	0.4	81.0	0	0	—	—	720
mayonnaise	1.1	2.2	0	2.2	80.0	70.0	0	—	—	718
French dressing	0.6	17.5	0	38.8	0	0	0	—	—	410
corn oil	0	0	0	0	100.0	0	0	—	—	884
safflower oil	0	0	0	0	100.0	0	0	—	—	884
olive oil	0	0	0	0	100.0	0	0	—	—	884
soybean oil	0	0	0	0	100.0	0	0	—	—	884
almonds	18.6	9.9	6.4	3.5	54.2	0	9.6	—	—	560
English walnuts	20.5	7.3	2.7	4.6	63.4	0	7.5	—	—	598
peanuts	26.0	9.5	6.1	3.4	49.7	0	9.3	—	—	546
pecans	9.2	7.4	6.3	1.1	71.2	0	7.2	—	—	659
bacon, crisp	25.0	0	0	0	55.0	100.0	0	—	—	603
butter*	0.6	0.7	0	0.7	81.0	280.0	0	—	—	717
sour cream*	2.7	3.7	0	3.7	19.3	20.0	0	—	—	196
cream, heavy*	7.6	2.7	0	2.7	35.3	111.0	0	—	—	353
lard*	0	0	0	0	100.0	95.0	0	—	—	902
peanut butter	26.3	18.8	12.1	6.7	48.8	0	0	—	—	575
vegetable shortening	0	0	0	0	100.0	0	0	—	—	884

not recommended but included for comparison purposes

Sodium Content of Food

Item	Food	Portion	Weight (grams)	Sodium (milligrams)
Beverages and Fruit Juices				
	Breakfast drink, instant:			
1	Citrus fruits	8 fl oz	240	14
2	Coffee	8 fl oz	240	2
	Fruit drinks, canned:			
3	Pineapple-grapefruit, canned	8 fl oz	240	80
	Fruit drinks, dehydrated, Reconstituted: Sweetened:			
4	Lemonade, canned	8 fl oz	240	50
5	Orange, canned	8 fl oz	240	35
	Tea:			
	Hot:			
6	Brewed	8 fl oz	240	1
Dairy Products				
	Cheese:			
	Natural:			
7	Blue	1 oz	28	396
8	Brick	1 oz	28	159
9	Camembert	1 oz	28	239
	Cheddar:			
10	Regular	1 oz	28	176
11	Low sodium	1 oz	28	6
	Cottage:			
12	Regular and low fat	4 oz	113	457
13	Dry curd, unsalted	4 oz	113	14
14	Cream	1 oz	28	84
15	Feta	1 oz	28	316
16	Gruyère	1 oz	28	95
	Mozzarella, from:			
17	Whole milk	1 oz	28	106
18	Part skim milk	1 oz	28	132
19	Muenster	1 oz	28	178
	Parmesan:			
20	Grated	1 oz	28	528
21	Provolone	1 oz	28	248
	Ricotta, made with:			
22	Whole milk	½ cup	124	104
23	Part skim milk	½ cup	124	155
24	Roquefort	1 oz	28	513
25	Swiss	1 oz	28	74

NOTE: Values taken from "The Sodium Content of Food," U.S. Dept. of Agriculture, *Home and Garden Bulletin #233.*

Sodium Content of Food (continued)

Item	Food	Portion	Weight (grams)	Sodium (milligrams)
	Pasteurized processed cheese:			
26	American	1 oz	28	406
27	Low sodium	1 oz	28	2
	Milk:			
	Fluid:			
28	Whole and low fat	1 cup	244	122
29	Whole, low sodium	1 cup	244	6
	Buttermilk, cultured:			
30	Salted	1 cup	245	257
	Canned:			
	Evaporated:			
31	Whole	1 cup	252	266
32	Sweetened, condensed	1 cup	306	389
	Dry:			
	Nonfat:			
33	Regular	½ cup	60	322
	Milk beverages:			
34	Chocolate	1 cup	250	149
	Milk desserts, frozen:			
	Ice cream:			
35	Chocolate	1 cup	133	75
	Ice milk:			
	Vanilla:			
36	Hardened	1 cup	131	105
37	Sherbet, orange	1 cup	193	89
	Milk desserts, other:			
	Puddings:			
	Butterscotch:			
38	Regular, whole milk	½ cup	148	245
39	Instant, whole milk	½ cup	149	445
	Chocolate:			
40	Regular, whole milk	½ cups	148	195
	Vanilla:			
41	Home recipe	½ cup	128	83
42	Regular, whole milk	½ cup	148	200
43	Instant, whole milk	½ cup	149	400
	Yogurt:			
	Plain:			
44	Regular	8 oz	227	105
45	Skim milk	8 oz	227	174

Eggs, Fish, Shellfish, Meat, Poultry and Related Products

	Eggs:			
46	Whole	1 egg	50	59
47	White	1 white	33	50

Sodium Content of Food (continued)

Item	Food	Portion	Weight (grams)	Sodium (milligrams)
	Fish:			
48	Bass, black sea, raw	3 oz	85	57
	Bluefish:			
49	Baked with butter	3 oz	85	87
50	Bonito, canned	3 oz	85	437
51	Haddock, breaded, fried	3 oz	85	150
52	Herring, smoked	3 oz	85	5,234
53	Mackerel, raw	3 oz	85	40
54	Ocean perch, fried	3 oz	85	128
	Salmon:			
55	Broiled with butter	3 oz	85	99
	Canned:			
	Salt added:			
56	Pink, canned	3 oz	85	443
57	Without salt added	3 oz	85	41
	Sardines, canned:			
58	Drained	3 oz	85	552
	Tuna, canned:			
	Light meat, chunk:			
59	Oil pack	3 oz	85	303
60	Water pack	3 oz	85	288
	White meat (Albacore):			
61	Chunk, low sodium	3 oz	85	34
	Solid:			
62	Oil pack	3 oz	85	384
63	Water pack	3 oz	85	309
	Shellfish:			
	Clams, raw:			
64	Hard	3 oz	85	174
	Crab:			
65	Canned, drained	3 oz	85	425
66	Steamed	3 oz	85	314
67	Lobster, boiled	3 oz	85	212
68	Mussels, raw	3 oz	85	243
	Oysters:			
69	Raw	3 oz	85	113
70	Fried	3 oz	85	174
71	Frozen	3 oz	85	323
	Scallops:			
72	Steamed	3 oz	85	225
	Shrimp:			
73	Raw	3 oz	85	137
74	Canned	3 oz	85	1,955

Sodium Content of Food (continued)

Item	Food	Portion	Weight (grams)	Sodium (milligrams)
	Meat:			
	Beef:			
75	Cooked, lean	3 oz	85	55
	Corned:			
76	Cooked	3 oz	85	802
77	Canned	3 oz	85	893
78	Dried, chipped	1 oz	28	1,219
79	Lamb, cooked, lean	3 oz	85	58
	Pork:			
	Cured:			
	Bacon:			
80	Cooked	2 slices	14	274
81	Canadian	1 slice	28	394
82	Ham	3 oz	85	1,114
83	Veal, cooked, lean	3 oz	85	69
	Organ meats:			
84	Kidney, beef, braised	1 oz	28	71
	Liver:			
85	Calf, fried	1 oz	28	33
	Poultry and game:			
	Chicken, roasted:			
86	Breast with skin	½ breast	98	69
87	Drumstick with skin	1 drumstick	52	47
	Duck, roasted, flesh			
88	and skin	½ duck	382	227
	Goose, roasted, flesh			
89	and skin	½ goose	774	543
	Turkey, small, roasted:			
90	Breast with skin	½ breast	344	182
91	Leg with skin	1 leg	245	195
	Sausages, luncheon meats, and spreads:			
	Bologna:			
92	Beef	1 slice	22	220
93	Braunschweiger	1 slice	28	324
94	Frankfurter	1 frankfurter	57	639
95	Knockwurst	1 link	68	687
96	Olive loaf	1 slice	21	312
97	Pepperoni	1 slice	6	122
	Salami:			
	Cooked:			
98	Dry or hard, pork	1 slice	10	226

Sodium Content of Food (continued)

Item	Food	Portion	Weight (grams)	Sodium (milligrams)
	Sausage:			
	Cooked:			
99	Pork	1 link	13	168
	Prepared main dishes:			
	Beef:			
	Chili con carne with beans, canned:			
100	Regular	1 cup	255	1,194
101	Low sodium	1 cup	335	100
	Dinners, frozen:			
102	Beef	1 dinner	312	998
103	Meat loaf	1 dinner	312	1,304
104	Goulash, canned	8 oz	227	1,032
	Hash, corned beef,			
105	canned	1 cup	220	1,520
106	Meatballs, Swedish	8 oz	227	1,880
	Pizza, frozen:			
107	With pepperoni	½ pie	195	813
	Pot pie:			
108	Frozen	1 pie	227	1,093
109	Ravioli, canned	7.5 oz	213	1,065
	Spaghetti, canned:			
110	And ground beef	7.5 oz	213	1,054
111	Stew, canned	8 oz	227	980
	Pork, sweet and sour			
112	canned	1 cup	275	1,968
	Turkey:			
113	Dinner, frozen	1 dinner	333	1,228
	Fast foods:			
114	Cheeseburger	1 each	111	709
115	Chicken dinner	1 portion	410	2,243
116	Fish sandwich	1 sandwich	164	882
	Hamburger:			
117	Regular	1 each	92	461
118	Jumbo	1 each	236	990
119	Taco	1 taco	75	401
Fruits				
	Apples:			
120	Raw or baked	1 apple	138	2
121	Dried, sulfured	8 oz	227	210
	Applesauce, canned:			
122	Sweetened	1 cup	250	6
123	With added salt	1 cup	250	68

Sodium Content of Food (continued)

Item	Food	Portion	Weight (grams)	Sodium (milligrams)
124	Banana, raw	1 banana	119	2
	Berries:			
	Blackberries (boysenberries)			
125	Raw	1 cup	144	1
126	Canned	1 cup	244	3
	Strawberries:			
127	Raw	1 cup	149	2
128	Frozen, sliced	1 cup	255	6
	Cherries:			
129	Raw	1 cup	150	1
130	Canned	1 cup	257	10
	Citrus:			
	Grapefruit:			
131	Raw	½ grapefruit	120	1
132	Cranberry, raw	1 cup	95	1
133	Cranberry sauce	1 cup	277	75
	Muskmelon:			
134	Cantaloupe	½ melon	272	24
	Peaches:			
135	Raw	1 peach	100	1
136	Canned	1 cup	256	15
	Pears:			
137	Raw	1 pear	168	1
138	Canned	1 cup	255	15
	Pineapple:			
139	Raw	1 cup	135	1
140	Canned	1 cup	255	7
141	Raisins, seedless	1 cup	145	17
Grain Products				
	Biscuits, baking powder:			
142	Regular flour	1 biscuit	28	175
143	Low sodium	1 biscuit	28	1
	Bread:			
144	Corn, homemade	1 oz	28	176
145	French	1 slice	23	116
146	Mixed grain	1 slice	23	138
147	Pita	1 loaf	64	132
	Rye:			
148	Regular	1 slice	25	139
149	Pumpernickel	1 slice	32	182
	White:			
150	Regular	1 slice	25	114
151	Low sodium	1 slice	23	7

Sodium Content of Food (continued)

Item	Food	Portion	Weight (grams)	Sodium (milligrams)
152	Whole wheat	1 slice	25	132
	Breakfast cereals:			
	Hot, cooked, in unsalted water:			
	Corn (hominy) grits:			
153	Regular	1 cup	236	1
154	Instant	¾ cup	177	354
	Cream of Wheat:			
155	Regular	¾ cup	184	2
156	Instant	¾ cup	184	5
157	Mix 'n' eat	¾ cup	184	250
	Oatmeal:			
158	Regular or quick	¾ cup	180	1
	Instant:			
159	Sodium added	¾ cup	180	283
	Ready-to-eat:			
	Bran cereals:			
160	All-Bran	⅓ cup	28	160
161	40% Bran	⅔ cup	28	251
162	100% Bran	½ cup	28	221
163	Raisin Bran	½ cup	28	209
164	Cheerios	1¼ cup	28	304
	Corn cereals:			
	Corn flakes:			
165	Low sodium	1¼ cup	28	10
166	Regular	1 cup	28	256
	Granola:			
167	Regular	¼ cup	34	61
168	No sodium added	¼ cup	34	16
	Rice cereals:			
169	Low sodium	1 cup	28	10
170	Puffed rice	2 cups	28	2
171	Rice Chex	1⅛ cup	28	238
172	Rice Krispies	1 cup	28	340
173	Special K	1¼ cup	28	265
174	Total	1 cup	28	359
	Wheat cereals:			
175	Puffed wheat	2 cups	28	2
176	Shredded wheat	1 biscuit	24	3
	Cakes, from mix:			
	Angel food:			
177	Regular	1/12 cake	56	134
178	Devil's food	1/12 cake	67	402
179	Pound	1/12 cake	55	171

Sodium Content of Food (continued)

Item	Food	Portion	Weight (grams)	Sodium (milligrams)
	Cookies:			
180	Brownies, iced	1 brownie	32	69
181	Chocolate chip	2 cookies	21	69
182	Ginger snaps	4 cookies	28	161
	Oatmeal:			
183	Plain	1 cookies	18	77
184	Vanilla wafer	6 cookies	24	53
	Crackers:			
185	Graham	1 cracker	7	48
186	Low sodium	1 cracker	4	1
187	Saltine	2 crackers	6	70
188	Pancakes, from mix	1 pancake	27	152
189	Pancake mix	1 cup	141	2,036
	Rice, cooked:			
190	Brown	1 cup	195	10
	White:			
191	Regular	1 cup	205	6
	Snacks:			
192	Potato chips	10 chips	20	200
	Pretzels:			
193	Regular twist	1 pretzel	6	101
194	Spaghetti, cooked	1 cup	140	2

Legumes and Nuts

Item	Food	Portion	Weight (grams)	Sodium (milligrams)
	Amonds			
195	Salted, roasted	1 cup	157	311
196	Unsalted, slivered	1 cup	115	4
	Beans:			
	Baked, canned:			
197	Boston style	1 cup	260	606
198	With or without pork	1 cup	260	928
	Dry, cooked:			
199	Lima	1 cup	192	4
	Cashews:			
200	Roasted in oil	1 cup	140	21
201	Dry roasted, salted	1 cup	140	1,200
202	Chestnuts	1 cup	160	10
	Filberts (hazelnuts),			
203	chopped	1 cup	115	2
	Peanuts:			
204	Dry roasted, salted	1 cup	144	986
205	Unsalted	1 cup	144	8

Sodium Content of Food (continued)

Item	Food	Portion	Weight (grams)	Sodium (milligrams)
	Peanut butter:			
206	Smooth or crunchy	1 tbsp	16	81
207	Low sodium	1 tbsp	16	1
208	Pecans	1 cup	118	1
209	Pistachios	1 cup	125	6
	Soybeans:			
210	Cooked	1 cup	180	4
211	Walnuts, English	1 cup	120	3
Soups				
212	Beef broth, cubed	1 cup	241	1,152
	Beef noodle:			
213	Dehydrated, with water	1 cup	251	1,041
	Chicken noodle:			
214	Dehydrated, with water	1 cup	252	1,284
	Chicken rice:			
215	Dehydrated, with water	1 cup	253	980
	Clam chowder, Manhattan,			
216	condensed, with water	1 cup	244	1,029
	Clam chowder, New England,			
	condensed:			
217	With water	1 cup	244	914
	Mushroom:			
218	Condensed, with milk	1 cup	248	1,076
219	Low sodium	1 cup	244	27
	Pea, green:			
220	Dehydrated, with water	1 cup	271	1,220
	Tomato:			
221	Dehydrated, with water	1 cup	265	943
222	Low sodium	1 cup	244	29
	Vegetable beef:			
223	Dehydrated, with water	1 cup	252	1,000
224	Low sodium	1 cup	244	51
Sugars and Sweets				
	Candy:			
225	Caramel	1 oz	28	74
	Chocolate:			
226	Bitter	1 oz	28	4
227	Milk	1 oz	28	28
228	Fudge, chocolate	1 oz	28	54
229	Mints, uncoated	1 oz	28	56
230	Peanut brittle	1 oz	28	145

Sodium Content of Food (continued)

Item	Food	Portion	Weight (grams)	Sodium (milligrams)
	Jams and Jellies:			
	Jam:			
231	Regular	1 tbsp	20	2
	Syrup:			
	Maple:			
232	Regular	1 tbsp	20	1
233	Imitation	1 tbsp	20	20
	Sugar:			
234	Brown	1 cup	220	66
235	Granulated	1 cup	200	2

Vegetables, Vegetable Juices and Salads

Item	Food	Portion	Weight (grams)	Sodium (milligrams)
	Artichokes:			
236	Hearts, frozen	3 oz	85	40
	Asparagus:			
237	Raw	1 spear	20	1
238	Frozen	4 spears	60	4
	Canned:			
239	Regular	4 spears	80	298
	Beans:			
	Lima:			
240	Cooked	1 cup	170	2
241	Frozen	1 cup	170	128
242	Canned	1 cup	170	456
243	Low sodium	1 cup	170	7
	Beets:			
244	Cooked	1 cup	170	73
	Canned:			
245	Sliced	1 cup	170	479
	Broccoli:			
246	Raw	1 stalk	151	23
	Carrots:			
247	Raw	1 carrot	72	34
	Frozen:			
248	Cut or whole	3.3 oz	94	43
	Canned:			
249	Regular	1 cup	155	386
250	Lettuce	1 cup	55	4
	Mushrooms:			
251	Raw	1 cup	70	7
252	Canned	2 oz	56	242
253	Parsley, raw	1 tbsp	4	2

Sodium Content of Food (continued)

Item	Food	Portion	Weight (grams)	Sodium (milligrams)
	Peas, green:			
254	Cooked	1 cup	160	2
	Frozen:			
255	Regular	3 oz	85	80
	Canned:			
256	Regular	1 cup	170	493
	Potatoes:			
257	Baked or boiled	1 medium	156	5
	Frozen:			
258	French fried	10 strips	50	15
259	Salted	2.5 oz	71	270
260	Canned	1 cup	250	753
261	Instant, reconstituted	1 cup	210	485
262	Au gratin	1 cup	245	1,095
	Spinach:			
263	Raw	1 cup	55	49
	Canned:			
264	Regular	1 cup	205	910
	Tomatoes:			
265	Raw	1 tomato	123	14
	Canned:			
266	Whole	1 cup	240	390
267	Stewed	1 cup	240	584
268	Low sodium	1 cup	240	16
	Tomato juice:			
269	Regular	1 cup	243	878
270	Low sodium	1 cup	243	9
271	Tomato paste	1 cup	258	77
272	Tomato sauce	1 cup	248	1,498
	Vegetables, mixed:			
273	Frozen	3.3 oz	94	45
274	Canned	1 cup	170	380

Condiments, Fats and Oils

Item	Food	Portion	Weight (grams)	Sodium (milligrams)
275	Baking powder	1 tsp	3	339
276	Baking soda	1 tsp	3	821
	Catsup:			
277	Regular	1 tbsp	15	156
278	Low sodium	1 tbsp	15	3
	Garlic:			
279	Powder	1 tsp	3	1
280	Salt	1 tsp	6	1,850

Sodium Content of Food (continued)

Item	Food	Portion	Weight (grams)	Sodium (milligrams)
281	Horseradish, prepared	1 tbsp	18	198
	Meat tenderizer:			
282	Regular	1 tsp	5	1,750
283	Low sodium	1 tsp	5	1
284	MSG (monosodium glutamate)	1 tsp	5	492
285	Mustard, prepared	1 tsp	5	65
	Olives:			
286	Green	4 olives	16	323
	Onion:			
287	Powder	1 tsp	2	1
288	Salt	1 tsp	5	1,620
289	Parsley, dried	1 tbsp	1	6
	Pickles:			
290	Dill	1 pickle	65	928
291	Sweet	1 pickle	15	128
292	Salt	1 tsp	5	1,938
	Sauces:			
293	A-1	1 tbsp	17	275
294	Barbecue	1 tbsp	16	130
	Chili:			
295	Regular	1 tbsp	17	227
296	Low sodium	1 tbsp	15	11
297	Soy	1 tbsp	18	1,029
298	Tabasco	1 tsp	5	24
299	Tartar	1 tbsp	14	182
300	Teriyaki	1 tbsp	18	690
301	Worcestershire	1 tbsp	17	206
	Fats, oils, and related products:			
	Butter:			
302	Regular	1 tbsp	14	116
303	Unsalted	1 tbsp	14	2
	Margarine:			
304	Regular	1 tbsp	14	140
305	Unsalted	1 tbsp	14	1
	Oil, vegetable, (includes			
306	corn, olive, and soybean)	1 tbsp	14	0
	Salad dressing:			
307	Blue cheese	1 tbsp	15	153
	French:			
303	Home recipe	1 tbsp	14	92
309	Bottled	1 tbsp	14	214
310	Dry mix, prepared	1 tbsp	14	253
311	Low sodium	1 tbsp	15	3

Sodium Content of Food (continued)

Item	Food	Portion	Weight (grams)	Sodium (milligrams)
	Italian:			
312	Bottled	1 tbsp	15	116
313	Dry mix, prepared	1 tbsp	14	172
314	Mayonnaise	1 tbsp	15	78
315	Russian	1 tbsp	15	133
	Thousand Island:			
316	Regular	1 tbsp	16	109

Bibliography

Alexander, S. "Newer Cardiovascular Drugs, Audio Digest, Internal Medicine." *Topics in Cardiology* 28: 1–4, 1981.

Alpert, J. S., and Rippe, J. M. *Manual of Cardiovascular Diagnosis and Therapy.* Boston: Little Brown & Company, 1982.

Altura, Burton. "Have We Sold Magnesium Short?" *Wellcome Trends in Cardiology*, Burroughs, Welcome Publishing, November 1982.

American Academy of Pediatrics Committee on Nutrition. "Salt Intake and Eating Patterns of Infants and Children in Relation to Blood Pressure." *Pediatrics* 53: 115–121, 1974.

American Heart Association, Central Committee. "Dietary fat and its relation to heart attacks and strokes." *Circulation* 23: 1961.

American Heart Association, Subcommittee on Diet & Hyperlipidemia, Council on Arteriosclerosis. "A Maximal Approach to the Dietary Treatment of the Hyperlipidemias: Diet A; Diet B." New York: American Heart Association, 1973.

American Heart Association. "The Value and Safety of Diet Modification to Control Hyperlipidemia in Childhood and Adolescence. A Statement for Physicians." Reprinted from *Circulation* 58:381A 1–6, 1978.

American Heart Association. *The American Heart Association Cookbook*, 3rd ed. New York: David McKay Company, 1975.

American Heart Association, Nutrition Committee of the Steering Committee for Medical and Community Programs. "Diet and Coronary Artery Disease—A Statement for Physicians and Other Health Professionals." (1978): pp. 1–7.

American Heart Association. *Heart Facts*, 1984, pp. 1–25.

American Heart Association, Nutrition Committee, Supplement to Guidelines for the Development of Nutrition Programs—1981. 1–34.

Anderson, J. W. "Effects of Carbohydrate Restriction & High Carbohydrate Diets on Men with Chemical Diabetes." *American Journal of Clinical Nutrition* 3: 402–8, 1977.

Anderson, J. W. *HCF—High Carbohydrate & Fiber—Diet Book*, New York: Aric Publishers, 1982.

Bachman, David S. "Group Smoking Deterrent Therapy." *General Practitioner* 30: 86, September 1964.

Bailar, J. C. "Cause and Effect in Epidemiology." *New England Journal of Medicine* 302: 1417–18, 1980.

Bain, C., Willett, W., Hennekens, C. H., Rosner, B., Belanger, C., and Speizer, E. E. "Use of postmenopausal hormones and risk of myocardial infarction." *Circulation* 64:42–6, 1981.

Bassler, T. In *The Marathon: Physiological, Medical, Epidemiological & Psychological Studies.* Edited by P. Milvy. New York: Academy of Science 1977, p. 579.

Baumberger, J. P. "Nicotine content of tobacco smoke." *Journal of Pharmacology and Experimental Therapy* 21: 35, 1923.

Baumgartner, M. A. *The Book of Whole Grains.* New York: St. Martin's Press, 1976.

Benson, H., Alexander, S., and Feldman, C. L. "Decreased Premature Ventricular Contractions Through Use of Relaxation Response in Patients with Stable Ischemic Heart Disease." *Lancet,* August 30, 1975, 380–82.

Benson, H. *The Relaxation Response.* New York: William Morrow & Company, 1975.

Benson, H. "Systemic Hypertension and the Relaxation Response." *New England Journal of Medicine* 296: 1152, 1977.

Berger, A., and Schaumberg, H. H. "More on Neuropathy from Pyridoxine Abuse." *New England Journal of Medicine* 311: 986–87, 1984.

Blair, S. N., Goodyear, N. N., Gibbons, L. W., and Cooper, K. H. "Physical Fitness and Incidence of Hypertension in Healthy Normotensive Men and Women." *Journal of the American Medical Association* 252:487–90, 1984.

Bottiger, L. E., Carlson, L. A., Hultman, E., and Romanus V. "Serum Lipids in Alcoholics." *Acta Medica Scandinavica* 199: 357–61, 1976.

Belfrage, P., Berg, B., Hägerstrand, I., Nillson-Ehle, P., Tornquist, H., & Wiebe, T. "Alterations of Lipid Metabolism in Healthy Volunteers During Longtime Ethanol Intake." *European Journal of Clinical Investigation* 7: 127–31, 1977.

Brown, W. J., Liebowitz, D., and Olness, M. *Cook to Your Heart's Content on a Low-Fat, Low-Salt Diet.* New York: Van Nostrand Reinhold Co., 1976.

Brunner, D. "Atherosclerosis, other vascular complications, and lipid pattern in diabetic Yemenite Jews." *Circulation* 21: 895, 1961.

Brunner, D. "Lipid pattern in Yemenite Jews and in Middle-aged coronary patients without increased total serum cholesterol." *Circulation* 24: 896, 1961.

Burkitt, D. P., Walker, A. R. P., and Painteir, N. S. "Dietary fiber and diseases." *Journal of American Medical Association* 229: 1068–74, 1974.

Bush, T., Cowan, L., Barrett-Connor, E., et al. "Reduction of all cause mortality in estrogen users: preliminary results from the Lipid Research Clinics (LRC) Program's follow-up study." *CVD Epidemiology Newsletter* (1982) 31:49.

Cambien, F., Richard, D. L., and Ducemetière, A. "Sports Activity, Paternal History and The Risk of Coronary Heart Disease." *New England Journal of Medicine* 303: 887, 1980.

Carlon, R. A., Ignani, E., Stewart, K., and Dorval, J. "Fire Deaths from Smoking." *New England Journal of Medicine* 301: 309, 1979.

Castelli, W. P., Doyle, J. T., Gordon, T., et al. "Alcohol & Blood Lipids: The Cooperative Lipoprotein Phenotyping Study." *Lancet* 2: 153–55, 1977.

Castelli, W. P., Garrison, R. J., Dawber, T. R., McNamara, P. M., Feinleib, M., and Kannel, W. B. "The Filter Cigarette and Coronary Heart Disease: The Framingham Study." *Lancet* 2: 109–13, 1981.

Castelli, W. P., Doyle, J. T., Gordon, T., Hames, C. G., Hortland, M. C., Hulley, S. B., Kagan, A., and Zukel, W. J. "HDL Cholesterol and Other Lipids in Coronary Heart Disease. The Cooperative Lipoprotein Phenotyping Study." *Circulation* 55: 767–72, 1977.

Chave, S. P. W., Morris, J. N., Moss, S., and Semmence, A. M. "Vigorous Exercise in Leisure Time and the Death Rate: A Study of Male Civil Servants." *Journal of Epidemiology Community Health* 32: 239–45, 1978.

Colgan, M. *Your Personal Vitamin Profile.* New York: Quill, 1982.

Colley, J. R. P., Holland, W. W., and Corkhill, R. T. "Influence of Passive Smoking and Parenteral Phlegm in Pneumonia and Bronchitis in Early Childhood." *Lancet* 2:1031, 1974.

Connor, W. E., and Connor, S. L. "The Dietary Treatment of Hyperlipidemia: Rationale, Technique and Efficacy." *Medical Clinics of North America* 66: 485–518, 1982.

Connor, W. E., Connor, S. L., Becker, N., et al. *The Best from the Family Heart Kitchens.* Portland, Ore.: Oregon; Health Sciences University Press, 1981.

Cressman, M. D., and Gifford, R. W. "Hypertension & Stroke." *Journal of American College of Cardiology* 1: 521–27, 1983.

Dahl, L. K. "Salt & Hypertension." *American Journal of Clinical Nutrition* 25: 231, 1972.

Davis, M., McKay, M., and Eshelman, E. R. *The Relaxation & Stress Reduction Workbook,* 2nd ed. Oakland, Calif.: New Harbinger Publications, 1982.

Dawber, T. R., and Kannel, W. B. "An epidemiologic study of heart disease." *Nutrition Reviews* 16:1, 1958.

Dawber, T. R., and Kannel, W. B. "Susceptibility to Coronary Heart Disease." *Modern Concepts in Cardiovascular Disease* 30: 7, 671, 1961.

Dawber, T. R., Moore, F. E., and Mann, G. V. "Coronary heart disease in the Framingham Study." *American Journal of Public Health* 47: 4–24, 1957.

Dawber, T. R., Kannel, W. B., Kayan, A., Donabedian, R. K., McNamara, P. M., and Pearsen, G. "Environmental Factors in Hypertension." In Stamler, J., Stamler, R., and Pullonen, T. N. *The Epidemiology of Hyptertension.* New York: Grune & Hutton, 1967, page 255.

Dobemeyer, D. J., Stine, R. A., Leier, C. V., Greenberg, R., and Schaal, S. F. "The Arrhythmogenic Effects of Caffeine in Human Beings." *New England Journal of Medicine* 308: 814–16, 1983.

Doisy, R. J., Streeten, D. H. P., Freiberg, J. M., and Schneider, A. J. "Chromium Metabolism in Man & Biochemical Effects." In *Trace Elements in Human Health & Disease,* volume II, edited by A. S. Prosad. New York: Academic Press, 1976.

Dunn, F. L. "Hyperlipidemia & Diabetes Symposium on Diabetes Mellitus." *Medical Clinics of North America* 66: 1347–60, 1982.

Dunn, F. "Hyptertension and Myocardial Infarction." *Journal of American College of Cardiology* 1: 528–32, 1983.

Dyer, A. R., Stamler, J., Paul, O., et al. "Alcohol Consumption, Cardiovascular Risk Factors, and Mortality in Two Chicago Epidemiologic Studies." *Circulation* 56: 1067–74, 1977.

Dyer, A., Garside, D., Stamler, R., et al. "Circulating cholesterol level and risk of death from cancer in men aged 40 to 69 years: experience of an international collaborative group." *Journal of American Medical Association* 248: 2853–59, 1982.

Editorial; "HDL & CHD," *Lancet* 131, July 17, 1976.

Ebler, H. A., and Gidez, L. I. "The Clinical Significance of the Plasma High Density Lipoproteins." *Medical Clinics of North America* 65: 431–40, 1982.

Ehnholm, C., Huttunen, J. K., Pietinen, P., Leino, W., Mutanen, M., Kostiainen, E., Pikkarainen, J., Dougherty, R., Ilacono, J., and Puska, P. "Effect of Diet on Serum Lipoproteins in a Population with a High Risk of Coronary Heart Disease." *New England Journal of Medicine* 307: 850–55, 1982.

Eliot, R. S. "Stress Management—Where Are We Now?" *Wellcome Trends in Cardiology* 2: 1–5, 1980.

Emergency Medicine. "For Diabetes, A Return to Innocence." September 15, 1979, pp. 27–54.

Enselberg, C. D. "Physical Activity and Coronary Heart Disease." *American Heart Journal* 80: 137–41, 1970.

Epstein, F. H. "Hyperglycemia, A Risk Factor in Coronary Heart Disease." *Circulation* 36: 609, 1967.

Ettinger, P. O.; Wu, C. F.; DeLaCruz, Jr.; et al. "Arrythmias and the 'Holiday Heart': Alcohol Associated Cardiac Rhythm Disorders." *American Heart Journal* 95: 555–62, 1978.

Fire in the United States: A Report of the National Fire Prevention & Control Administration. Washington, D.C.: National Fire Prevention & Control Administration, 1978.

Food and Drug Administration. "Risk of Myocardial Infarction in Users of Oral Contraceptives." *FDA Drug Bulletin* 5: 10, 1975.

Fox, Samuel M. III. "Sex à la Debussy." *Clinical Trends in Cardiology,* September/October 1978: 5.

Frank, C. W., Weinblatt, E., Shapiro, S., and Sager, R. V. "Physical Inactivity as a Lethal Factor in Myocardial Infarction Among Men." *Circulation* 34: 1022–33, 1966.

French, A. J., and Dock, W. "Fatal coronary arteriosclerosis in young soldiers." *Journal of American Medical Association* 124: 1232–37, 1944.

Friedman, M., and Rosenman, R. *Type A Behavior and Your Heart.* New York: Alfred A. Knopf, 1974.

Ginter, E. O., Cerna, O., Budlovsky, J., Bulaz, V., Hruba, F., Roch, V., and Sasko, E. "Effect of ascorbic acid on plasma cholesterol in Humans in a Long Term Experience." *International Journal of Vitamins & Nutrition Research* 47: 123–34, 1977.

Glinsmann, W. H., and Mertz, W. "Effect of Trivalent Chromium on Glucose Tolerance." *Metabolic Clinical Experiments* 15: 510–20, 1966.

Glomset, J. A. "Fish, Fatty Acids, and Human Health" (editorial). *New England Journal of Medicine* 312: 1253–1254, 1985.

Glueck, C. J., and Connor, W. E. "Diet—Coronary Heart Disease Relationships Reconnoitered." *American Journal of Clinical Nutrition* 31: 727–37, 1978.

Glueck, C. J., McGill, H. C., Lauer, R. M., et al. *The Value and Safety of Diet Modification to Control Hyperlipidemia in Childhood and Adolescence: A Statement for Physicians.* Dallas: American Heart Association, 1978.

Goldberg, L., Elliot, D. L., Schutz, R. W., and Kloster, F. E. "Changes in Lipid and Lipoprotein Levels After Weight Training." *Journal of American Medical Association* 252: 504–06, 1984.

Goodman, A. G., Gilman, L. S., and Gilman, A. *Goodman & Gilman's The Pharmacological Basis of Therapeutics.* New York: Macmillan, 1980.

Gordon, T., Kannel, W. B., and McGee, D. "Death and Coronary Attacks in Men after Giving up Cigarette Smoking: 'A Report From the Framingham Study.'" *Lancet* 2: 1345–48, 1974.

Graboys, T. B., and Lown, B. "Coffee, Arrhythmias and Common Sense"—Editorial. *New England Journal of Medicine* 308: 835–37, 1983.

Greenberg, L. D., and Rinehart, J. F. "Plasma Cholesterol Levels of Cholesterol Fed, Control and Pyridoxine Deficient Monkeys." *Proceedings of the Society of Experimental Biology and Medicine* 76: 580, 1951.

Grundy, S. M. "Hypertriglyceridemia: Mechanisms, Clinical Significance and Treatment." *Medical Clinics of North America* 66: 519–35, 1982.

Hamilton, W., Hammermeister, K. E., DeRorien, T. A., Zia, M. S., and Dodge, H. T. "Effect of Coronary Artery Bypass Grafting on Subsequent Hospitalization." *American Journal of Cardiology* 51: 353–60, 1983.

Hammond, E. C., Garfinkel, L., Seidman, H., and Lew, E. A. "Some Recent Findings Concerning Cigarette Smoking." In *Origin of Human Cancer, Book A. Incidence of Cancer in Humans* (Cold Spring Harbor Conferences on Cell Proliferation Vol. 4), H. H. Hiatt, J. P. Watson, and J. A. Whisten, Eds. New York: Cold Spring Harbor Laboratory, 1977, pp. 101–12.

Hartung, G. H.; Foreyt, J. P.; Mitchell, R. E.; Vlasek, I.; and Gotto, A. M., Jr. "Relation of Diet to High Density Lipoprotein Cholesterol in Middle Aged Marathon Runners, Joggers and Inactive Men." *New England Journal of Medicine* 302: 357–61, 1980.

Hartz, A. J., Anderson, A. J., Brooks, H. L., Manley, J. C., Parent, G. T., and Barboriak, J. J. "The Association of Smoking With Cardiomyopathy." *New England Journal of Medicine* 311: 1201–06, 1984.

Haskell, W. L.; Camargo, C., Jr.; Williams, P. T.; Vranizan, K. M.; Krauss, R. M.; Lindgren, F. T.; and Wood, P. D. "The Effect of Cessation & Resumption of Moderate Alcohol Intake in Serum High Density Lipoprotein Subfraction: A Controlled Study." *New England Journal of Medicine* 310: 805–10, 1984.

Havel, R. J. "Approach to the Patient with Hyperlipidemia." *Medical Clinics of North America* 66: 319–33, 1982.

Haynes, S. G., Feinleib, M., Levine, S., Scotch, N., and Kannel, W. B. "The Relationship of Psychosocial Factors to Coronary Heart Disease in the Framingham Study. II. Prevalence of Coronary Heart Disease." *American Journal of Epidemiology* 107: 384–402, 1978.

Heiss, G., Johnson, N. J., Reiland, S., Davis, C. E., and Tyroler, H. A. "The epidemiology of plasma high-density lipoprotein cholesterol levels: the Lipid Research Clinics Prevalence Study Summary." *Circulation* 62 (Suppl 4): IV–116–36, 1980.

Hellerstein, H. K., and Friedman, E. H. "Sexual Activity and the Post Coronary Patient." *Cardiac Rehabilitation* 3: 43–46, 1972.

Henze, K., Bucci, A., Signoretti, P., Menotti, A., and Ricci, G. "Alcoholic Intake and Coronary Risk Factors in a Population Group of Rome." *Nutrition Metabolism* 21 (Suppl. 1): 157–59, 1977.

Holmes, T. H., and Rahe, R. H. "The Social Readjustment Rating Scale." *Journal of Psychosomatic Research* 11: 213–18, 1967.

Holmes, T. H., and Holmes, T. S. "How Change Can Make Us Ill in Stress." *Blue Print for Health* 25: 66–76, 1974.

Hubert, H., Feinleib, M., McNamara, P. M., and Castelli, W. P. "Obesity as an Independent Risk Factor for Cardiovascular Disease in Framingham." Abstract 88. *CVD Epidemiology Newsletter* 31: 39. Council on Epidemiology, American Heart Association, 1982.

Hulley, S. B., Rosenman, R. H., Bowol, R. D., et al. "Epidemiology as a Guide to Clinical Decisions: The Association between Triglyceride and Coronary Heart Disease." *New England Journal of Medicine* 302: 1383, 1980.

Hurst, J. W., Logue, R. B., Schlant, R. C., and Wenger, N. K. *The Heart, Arteries and Veins.* New York: McGraw-Hill Book Company, Blakiston Publishing, 1978.

Hypertension Detection & Follow-up Program Cooperative Group. "The Effect and Treatment on Mortality in 'Mild Hypertension.' " *New England Journal of Medicine* 307: 926–80, 1982.

Ismail-Beigc, F., Reinhold, J. G., Faradji, B., and Abadc, P. "Effects of Cellulose added to diets of low and high fiber content upon the Metabolism of Calcium, Magnesium, Zinc & Phosphorous by man." *Journal of Nutrition* 107: 510–18, 1977.

Jenkins, W. C. "Heredity, Diet and Coronary Heart Disease, III." *Medical Journal* 120: 77–78, 1961.

Jenkins, D. J. A., Gaff, D. V., Leeds, A. R., Alberti, K. G. M. M., Wolever, T. M. S., Gassall, M. A., and Hockaday, T. D. R. "Unabsorbable Carbohydrate and Diabetes: Decreased postprandial hyperglycemia." *Lancet* 2: 172–74, 1976.

Jenkins, D. J. A., Leeds, A. R., Gassull, M. A., Cochet, B., and Albert, K. G. M. M. "Decrease in postprandial insulin and glucose concentrations by guar and pectin." *Annals of Internal Medicine* 86: 20–23, 1977.

Jick, H., Dinan, B., and Rothman, K. J. "Non Contraceptive Estrogens and Non Fatal Myocardial Infarction." *Journal of American Medical Association* 239 (14): 1407–08, 1978.

Kannel, W. B. "Cardiovascular Sequelae of Hypertension." *Work Up: Hypertension* 1: 3–15, 1977.

Kannel, W. B. "Coffee, Cocktails and Coronary Candidates." *New England Journal of Medicine* 297: 443, 1977.

Kannel, W. B., and Thom, T. J. "Implications of the Recent Decline in Cardiovascular Mortality." *Cardiovascular Medicine* (September): 983–97, 1979.

Kannel, W. B. "Some Lessons in Cardiovascular Epidemiology from Framingham." *American Journal of Cardiology* 37: 269, 1976.

Kannel, W. B., McGee, D., and Gordon, T. "A General Cardiovascular Risk Profile: The Framingham Study." *American Journal of Cardiology* 38: 46–51, 1976.

Kaufman, D., Helmrich, S. P., Rosenberg, L., Miettinen, O. S., and Shapiro, S. "Nicotine and Carbon Monoxide Content of Cigarette Smoke and The Risk of Myocardial Infarction in Young Men." *New England Journal of Medicine* 308: 409–13, 1983.

Keys, A. "Is Overweight a Risk Factor for Coronary Heart Disease?" *Cardiovascular Medicine* (December): 1233–43, 1979.

Keys, M., Keys, A. *The Benevolent Bean.* New York: Farrar, Straus & Giroux, 1972.

Konishi, F. "Food Energy Equivalents of Various Activities." *Journal of American Dietetic Association* 46: 186–88, 1965.

Krauss, R. M. "Regulation of High Density Lipoprotein Levels." *Medical Clinics of North America* 65: 403–30, 1982.

Kromhout, D., Bosschieter, E. B., and De Lezenne Coulander. "Cor: The Inverse Relation Between Fish Consumption and 20 Year Mortality from Coronary Heart Disease." *New England Journal of Medicine* 312: 1205–1209, 1985.

Kuller, W. H. "Epidemiology of Cardiovascular Diseases: Current Perspectives." *American Journal of Epidemiology* 104: 425, 1976.

Lee, T. H., Hoover, R. L., Williams, J. D., Sperling, R. I., Ravalese, J., III, Spur, B. W., Robinson, D. R., Corey, E. J., Lewis, R. A., and Austen, K. F. "Effect of Dietary Enrichment with Eicosapenaenoic and Docpsahexanoic Acids on *in vitro* Neutrophil and Monocyte Leukotriene Generation and Neutrophil Function." *New England Journal of Medicine* 312: 1217–1224, 1985.

Levy, R. I. "All You've Wanted to Know About HDL." *Wellcome Trends in Cardiology* 1: 4–5, 1979.

Lipid Research Clinics Program. The Lipid Research Clinics Coronary Primary Prevention Trial Results, Part 1. "Reduction in Incidence of Coronary Artery Disease." *Journal of the American Medical Association* 251: 351–64, 1984.

Lipid Research Clinics Program. The Lipid Research Clinics Coronary Primary Prevention Trial Results, Part 2. "The Relationship of Reduction in Incidence of Coronary Artery Disease to Cholesterol Lowering." *Journal of the American Medical Association* 251: 365–74, 1984.

Luce, G. G., and Peper, E. "Learning How to Relax." *Stress* 25: 84–94, 1974.

McGee, D. "Probability of Developing Certain Cardiovascular Diseases, in 8 years at specific value of some characteristics." *The Framingham Study*, edited by Kannel & Gordon, Section 28. Washington, D.C.: U.S. Government Printing Office, 1973.

McGee, D., and Gordon, T. "The results of the Framingham Study applied to four other U.S. based epidemiological studies of cardiovascular disease." Section 31. Washington, D.C.: Department of Health, Education and Welfare Publication No. 76 (National Institute of Health): 1083, 1976.

McKay, M., Davis, M., and Fanning, P. *Thoughts & Feelings, The Art of Cognitive Stress Intervention.* Richmond, Va.: New Harbinger Publications, 1981.

MacMahon, B., Trichopoulous, D., Cole, P., and Brown, J. "Cigarette Smoking and Urinary Estrogen." *New England Journal of Medicine* 307: 1062–64, 1982.

Mann, J. I., and Inman, W. H. W. "Oral Contraceptives & Death from Myocardial Infarction." *British Medical Journal* 2: 245–48, 1975.

Mann, J. I., Inman, W. H. W., and Thorogood, O. L. "Oral Contraceptive Use in older women and fatal myocardial infarction." *British Medical Journal* 2: 445–47, 1976.

Mann, J., and the Oxford Dietetic Group. *The Diabetics Diet Book: A New High Fiber*

Eating Program. New York: Arco Publishing, 1982.

Mann, J. I., Vassey, M. P., Thorogood, M., and Doll, R. "Myocardial Infarction in Young Women with Special Reference to Oral Contraceptives." *British Medical Journal* 2: 241–45, 1975.

Margolis, J. R., Kannel, W. S., Feinlieb, M., Dauber, T. R., and McNamara, P. M. "Clinical features of unrecognized Myocardial Infarction—Silent and Symptomatic—18 year follow-up." The Framingham Study *American Journal of Cardiology* 32: 1–7, 1973.

Martin, J. L., Wilson, J. R., Kleaveland, J. P., et al. "Effects of Cigarette Smoking on Systemic and Coronary Sinus Thromboxane and Prostacyclin Concentrations (abstr.)." *Circulation* 68 (Suppl. III): 3–165, 1983.

Masters, W. H., and Johnson, V. E. *Human Sexual Response.* Boston: Little Brown & Company, 1966.

Mayer, J. "Pediatric Arteriosclerosis, The Overlooked Beginnings of the National Epidemic." *Medical Opinion* (May 1974) Code 1F: 26.

Meade, T. W., Greenberg, G., Thompson, S. G. "Progestogens and cardiovascular reactions associated with oral contraceptives and a comparison of the safety of 50- and 30-mg. oestrogen preparations." *British Medical Journal* 280: 1157–61, 1980.

Meichenbaum, D., and Cameron, R. In M. J. Mahoney and C. E. Thorensen. *Self Control: Power to the Person.* Monterey, Calif.: Brooks/Cole Publishing, 1974.

Metropolitan Life Insurance Company. *Widows Increasing in Number.* Statistical Bulletin 39, Nov. 1958.

Metropolitan Life Insurance Company. "1983 Metropolitan Height and Weight Tables." *Statistical Bulletin* 64: 3–9, Jan.–June 1983.

Mikhailidis, D. P., Jeremy, J. Y., Barradas, M. A., Green, N., and Dandona, P. "Effect of Ethanol on Vascular Prostacyclin (Prostaglandin I synthesis, platelet aggregation and platelet thromboxane release." *British Medical Journal* 287: 1495–98, 1983.

Mikhailidis, D. P., Jenkins, W. J., Jeremy, J. Y., Barradas, M. A., and Dandona, P. "Ethanol and Arterial Disease (Correspondence)." *New England Journal of Medicine* 311: 537–38, 1984.

Miranda, P. M., and Horowitz, D. L. "High Fiber Diets in the Treatment of Diabetes Mellitus." *Annals of Internal Medicine* 88: 482–86, 1978.

Morgan, R. R. "Heart Disease and Alcoholism." *Circulation* 24: 1001, October 1961.

Morgan, T., Myers, J., and Carney, S. "Salt Restriction and Hypertension." *Practical Cardiology* 6: 37–41, 1980.

Morris, J. N., Heady, J. A., Raffle, C. A. B., Roberts, C. G., and Parks, J. W. "Coronary heart disease and physical activity of work." *Lancet* 2: 1111, 1953.

Morrison, S. C. "Occupational mortality in Scotland." *British Journal of Industrial Medicine* 14: 130, 1957.

Morris, J. N., Pattison, D. C., Gardner, M. J., and Raffle, P. A. B. "Incidence and Prediction of Ischemic Heart Disease in London Busmen." *Lancet* 2: 553–59, 1966.

Morris, J. N., Chave, S. P. W., Adam, C., Sirey, C., Epstein, L., and Sheehan, D. J. "Vigorous Exercise in Leisure Time and the Incidence of Coronary Heart Disease." *Lancet* 2: 553–59, 1973.

National Academy of Science, Food and Nutrition Board. *Toward Healthful Diets,* 1980.

National Center for Health Statistics. *Chartbook for the Conference on The Decline in Coronary Heart Disease.* August 1978.

National Center for Health Statistics, Monthly Vital Statistics Report., Vol. 27 #1, April 18, 1978.

National Diabetes Advisory Board. *The Prevention and Treatment of Five Complications of Diabetes.* Atlanta: U.S. Dept. of Health & Human Services/Public Health Service/Centers for Disease Control, 1983.

National Research Council, Food & Nutrition Board. *Recommended Dietary Allowances,* 9th ed. Washington, D.C.: National Academy of Sciences, 1980.

Nicod, P., Rehr, R., Winniford, M. D., Campbell, W. B., Firth, B. G., and Hillis, L. D.

"Acute Systemic and Coronary Hemodynamic and Serological Responses to Cigarette Smoking in Long-Term Smokers with Atherosclerotic Coronary Artery Disease." *Journal of the American College of Cardiology* 4: 964–71, 1984.

Oberleas, D., and Prasad, A. S. "Factors Affecting Zinc Homeostasis." In A. S. Prasad, ed., *Trace Elements in Human Health & Disease*. New York: Academic Press, 1976.

Ostrander, L. D., Jr.; Francis, T., Jr.; Haynes, N. S.; et al. "The Relationship of Cardiovascular Disease to Hyperglycemia." *Annals of Internal Medicine* 62: 1188, 1965.

Paffenbarger, R. S., Jr.; and Hale, W. E. "Work Activity and Coronary Heart Mortality." *New England Journal of Medicine* 293: 545–50, 1975.

Paffenbarger, R. S., Jr.; Wing, A. L.; and Hyde, R. T. "Physical Activity As An Index of Heart Attack Risk in College Alumni." *American Journal of Epidemiology* 108: 161–75, 1978.

Paffenbarger, R. S., and Hyde, R. T. "Exercise as Protection Against Heart Attack." Editorial, *New England Journal of Medicine* 30: 1026–27, 1980.

Paffenbarger, R. S., Hyde, R. T., Wing, A. C., and Steinmetz, C. H. "A Natural History of Athleticism and Cardiovascular Health." *Journal of the American Medical Association* 252: 491–95, 1984.

Page, L., Damon, A., and Moellering, R. "Antecedents of cardiovascular disease in six Solomon Island societies." *Circulation* 49: 1132–46, 1974.

Patterson, R. E., Horowitz, S. F., Eng., C., Meller, J., Goldsmith, M. D., Pichard, A. D., Halgash, D. A., Herman, M. V., and Gorlin, R. "Can Nominal Exercise Test Criteria Identify Patients with Left Main or 3-Vessel Coronary Disease after a Fresh Myocardial Infarction." *American Journal of Cardiology* 51: 361–77, 1983.

Persson, I., Raby, K., Fonss-bech, P., and Jensen, E. "Effect of Prolonged bran administration on serum levels of cholesterol, ionized calcium and iron in the elderly." *Journal of American Geriatric Society* 24: 334–35, 1976.

Phillipson, B. E., Rothrock, D. W., Connor, W. E., Harris, W. S., and Illingworth, R. "Reduction of Plasma Lipids, Lipoproteins and Apoproteins by Dietary Fish Oils in Patients with Hypertriglyceridemia." *New England Journal of Medicine* 312: 1210–1216, 1985.

Pooling Project Research Group. "Relationship of Blood Pressure, Serum cholesterol, Smoking habits relative to weight & ECG abnormalities to incidence of major coronary events: Final Report of the Pooling Project." *Journal of Chronic Diseases* 31: 261, 1978.

Prasad, A. S. *Trace Elements in Health and Disease*, vol. II, pp. 79–104. New York: Academic Press, 1976.

Prasad, A. S. *Trace Elements & Iron in Human Metabolism*. New York: Plenum Medical Book Co., 1978.

Rechnitzer, P. A., Cunningham, D. A., Andrew, G. M., Buck, C. W., et al. "Relation of Exercise to the Recurrence Rate of Myocardial Infarction in Men." *American Journal of Cardiology* 51: 65–69, 1983.

Reinhold, J. G., Nasr, K., Lahimgarzadeh, A., and Hedayati, H. "Effects of purified phytate & phytate-rich bread upon metabolism of zinc, calcium, phosphorous & nitrogen in man." *Lancet* 1: 283–88, 1973.

Reinhold, J. G., Faradji, B., Abadi, P., and Ismail-Beigi, F. "Decreased absorption of calcium, magnesium, zinc & phosphorous by humans due to increased fiber and phosphorous consumption as wheat bread." *Journal of Nutrition* 106: 493–503, 1976.

Riales, R., and Albrink, M. "Effect of Chromium Chloride Supplementation on glucose tolerance & serum lipids including high-density lipoprotein of adult men." *American Journal of Clinical Nutrition* 34: 2670–78, 1981.

Roberts, W. B., and Strong, J. P. "Atherosclerosis in Persons with Hypertension and Diabetes Mellitus." *Lab Investigation* 18: 538, 1968.

Robbins, S. L., and Cotran, R. S. *Pathological Basis of Disease*. Philadelphia: W. B. Saunders Co., 1979.

Rosenman, R. H., Brand, R. J., Schultz, R. I., and Friedman, M. "Multivariate prediction of coronary heart disease during 8.5 year follow-up in the Western Collaborative Group Study." *American Journal of Cardiology* 37: 903, 1976.

Royal College of Physicians. "Smoking or Health: A Report of the Royal College of Physicians." Kent, U.K.: Pitman Medical Publishing Co., Ltd. 1977, p. 103.

Rudman, D., and Williams, P. J. "Megadose Vitamins: Use and Misuse." *New England Journal of Medicine* 309: 488–89, 1983.

Russek, H. I. "Role of Emotional Stress in the Etiology of Clinical Coronary Heart Disease." *Diseases of the Chest* 52: 1–9, 1967.

Schroeder, H. A. "Relations Between Hardness of Water and Death Rates from Certain Chronic and Degenerative Diseases in the United States." *Journal of Chronic Diseases* 12: 586–91, 1960.

Schroeder, H. A., and Balassa, J. J. "Influence of Chromium, Cadmium & Lead in rat aortic lipids and circulating cholesterol." *American Journal of Physiology* 209: 433–37, 1965.

Seelig, M. S. "Human Requirements of Magnesium: factors that increase needs." Presented at International Symposium on Magnesium Deficit in Human Pathology, Vittel, France, May 9–15, 1971.

Shaumburg, H., Kaplan, J., Windebank, A., Vick, N., Rasmus, S., Pleasure, D., and Brown, M. J. "Sensory Neuropathy from Pyridoxine Abuse: A New Megavitamin Syndrome." *New England Journal of Medicine* 309: 445–54, 1983.

Skelelle, R. B., MacMillan-Shyrock, A., Paul, O., Lepper, M., Stamler, J., Liu, S., and Raynor, W. J. "Diet, Serum Cholesterol and Death from Coronary Heart Disease— The Western Electric Study." *New England Journal of Medicine* 304: 65–69, 1981.

Slone, D., Shapiro, S., Kaufman, D. W., Rosenberg, L., Miettinen, O. S., and Stotley, P. D. "Risk of Myocardial Infarction in Relation to Current and Discontinued Use of Contraceptives." *New England Journal of Medicine* 305: 420–24, 1981.

Sloane, D., Shapiro, S., Rosenberg, L., et al. "Relation of Cigarette Smoking to Myocardial Infarction in Young Women." *New England Journal of Medicine* 298 (23): 1273–76, 1978.

Stamler, J., Farinaro, E., McJonnier, L. M., Itall, Y., Moss, D., and Stamler, R. "Prevention and Control of Hypertension by Nutritional Hygienic Means." *Journal of American Medical Association* 243: 1819–23, 1980.

St. Leger, A. S., Cochrane, A. L., and Moore, F. "Factors associated with Cardiac Mortality in Developed Countries with Particular Reference to the Consumption of Wines." *Lancet* I: 1017, 1979.

Stadel, B. V. "Oral Contraceptives and Cardiovascular Disease, Part I." *New England Journal of Medicine* 305: 612–18, 1981.

Stadel, B. V. "Oral Contraceptives and Cardiovascular Disease, Part II." *New England Journal of Medicine* 305: 672–77, 1981.

Staub, H. W., Reussner, G., and Thiessen, R. T. J. "Serum Cholesterol Reduction by Chromium in Hypercholesterolemic rats." *Science* 166: 746–47, 1969.

Strong, J. P., and McGill, H. C. "The Pediatric Aspects of Atherosclerosis." *Journal of Atherosclerosis Research* 9: 251, 1969.

Taylor, C. B., Cox, G. E., and Trueheart, R. E. "Reversibility of Atherosclerosis Ill." *Medical Journal* 119: February, 1961.

Trowell, H. C. "Dietary fiber Hypothesis of the Etiology of Diabetes Mellitus." *Diabetes* 24: 762–65, 1975.

Tzagournis, M. "A Deadly Duo: Hypertension and Diabetes Mellitus." *Consultant*, September, 1981, 247–55.

U.S. Department of Agriculture by Catherine Adams. *Nutritive Value of American Foods In Common Units.* Agricultural Handbook #456. Washington, D.C.: Agriculture Research Service, November, 1975.

U.S. Department of Agriculture, Science & Education. *Administration and Human Nutri-*

tion, Ideas for Better Eating. Washington, D.C.: U.S. Government Printing Office, January 1981.

U.S. Department of Health, Education & Welfare. *Smoking and Health 1979.* Report of the Surgeon General. Washington, D.C.: U.S. Government Printing Office.

U.S. Surgeon General. *The Health Consequences of Smoking: Cardiovascular Disease—A Report of the Surgeon General.* U.S. Dept. of Health and Human Services, 1983.

University Group Diabetes Program. "Supplementary Report on Nonfatal Events in patients treated with tolbutamide." *Diabetes* 25: 1129–53 (supplement 6), 1976.

University Group Diabetes Program. "A Study of the Effects of Hypoglycemic Agents on Vascular Complications in Patients with Adult Onset Diabetes." *Diabetes* 19: 747–830 (supplement 2), 1970.

Veterans Administration Cooperative Study Group On Antihypertensive Agents. "Effects of Treatment on Morbidity in Hypertension: II Results in Patients with Diastolic Blood Pressure Averaging 90–114 mm. Hg." *Journal of American Medical Association* 213: 1143, 1970.

Wallace, R. B., Hoover, J. J., Sandler, D., Rifkind, B. M., and Tyroler, H. A. "Altered plasma-lipids associated with oral contraceptive or estrogen consumption: the Lipid Research Clinics Program." *Lancet* 2: 11–14, 1977.

Wallentin, L., and Larsson-Cohn, U. "Metabolic and hormonal effects of post-menopausal estrogen replacement treatment. II Plasma lipids." *Acta Endocrinol* (Copenh) 86: 597–607, 1977.

Weinberg, S. L. "The Patient with Heart Disease and the Cardiovascular Physician & Surgeon." *Journal of American College of Cardiology* 1: 6–12, 1983.

Willet, W., Hennekens, C. H., Siegel, A. J., Adner, M. M., and Castelli, W. P. "Alcohol Consumption & High Density Lipoprotein Cholesterol in Marathon Runners." *New England Journal of Medicine* 303: 1159–61, 1980.

Wilson, P. W., Garrison, R. J., Castelli, W. P., Feinleib, M., McNamara, P. M., Kannel, W. B. "Prevalence of coronary heart disease in the Framingham Offspring Study: role of lipoprotein cholesterols." *American Journal of Cardiology* 46: 649–54, 1980.

Wood, P. D., and Haskell, W. L. "The Effect of Exercise in Plasma High Density Lipoproteins." *Lipids* 14: 417–27, 1979.

Xavier, Pi-Sunyer. "Fiber: What's in it For You." *Diabetes Forecast,* May–June 1983, pp. 40–42

Yano, K., Rhoads, G. G., and Kagan, A. "Coffee, Alcohol & Risk of Coronary Heart Disease Among Japanese Men Living in Hawaii." *New England Journal of Medicine* 297: 405–19, 1978.

Zugibe, F. T., and Brown, K. D. "Lipid and Acid Polysaccharide Relationship in Human Aortas." *Circulation* 18: 804, 1958.

Zugibe, F. T., and Brown, K. D. "Histochemistry of the Cerebral Arteries." *Circulation* 20: 971, 1959.

Zugibe, F. T., and Brown, K. D. "Histochemical Studies of Atherogenesis: Human Aortas." *Circulation Research* 8: 287, 1960.

Zugibe, F. T., and Brown, K. D. "Histochemistry of the Coronary Arteries." *Circulation* 21: 654, 1960.

Zugibe, F. T., and Brown, K. D. "Histochemical Studies in Atherogenesis: Human Cerebral Arteries." *Circulation Research* 9: 820: 1961.

Zugibe, F. T., Bourke, D. W., and Brown, K. D. "A Plastic Injection Method for Post-Mortem Assessment of the Coronary Arteries: A Preliminary Report." *American Journal of Clinical Pathology* 35: 563, 1961; Tech. Bulletin 31: 77, 1961.

Zugibe, F. T. "The Relationship Between the Chonroitin Sulfates and Collagen in Human Arteries with Aging." *Journal of Gerontology* 16: 392, 1961.

Zugibe, F. T., and Fink, M. L. "Evaluation of Histochemical and Histologic Methods Used in Cardiovascular Research." *Circulation* 24: 1108, 1961.

Zugibe, F. T., and Fink, M. L. "Histochemical Studies of the Coronary Arteries and Aortas of the Minipig." *Circulation* 24: 1108, 1961.

Zugibe, F. T. "The Demonstration of the Individual Acid Mucopolysaccharides in Human Aortas, Coronary Arteries and Cerebral Arteries. I. The Methods." *Journal of Histochemistry and Cytochemistry* 10: 441–47, 1962.

Zugibe, F. T. "The Demonstration of the Individual Acid Mucopolysaccharides in Human Aortas, Coronary Arteries and Cerebral Arteries. II. Identification and Significance with Aging." *Journal of Histochemistry and Cytochemistry* 10: 448–61, 1962.

Zugibe, F. T. *Eat, Drink and Lower Your Cholesterol.* New York: McGraw-Hill Publishing Co., 1963.

Zugibe, F. T. "Histochemical Studies in Coronary Atherogenesis: Comparison with Aortic and Cerebral Atherogenesis." *Circulation Research* 3: 401–09, 1963.

Zugibe, F. T., and Vester, J. W. "Coronary Stenosis and Myocardial Enzyme Loss." *Circulation* 28: 828–29, 1963.

Zugibe, F. T.; Conley, T.; and Bell, P., Jr. "Grading Coronary Stenosis." *Circulation* 29: 33, 1964.

Zugibe, F. T., and Conley, T. "A Low Temperature Metal Alloy for Making Rapid Casts of Blood Vessels, Aortic Valves and Atherosclerotic Impressions of Opened Arteries." *Archives of Pathology* 77: 558, 1964.

Zugibe, F. T.; Bell, P., Jr.; and Conley, T. "Radiopaque Plastic Injection Technique for Assessing Coronary Stenosis and Collateralization at Autopsy." *Circulation* 29: 32–33, 1964.

Zugibe, F. T. "The Natural History of Vascular Change." In *Clinical Features of the Aging Patient.* Edited by J. T. Freeman. Philadelphia: Charles T. Thomas Publishing Co., 1965, pp. 91–102.

Zugibe, F. T.; Conley, T.; Bell, P., Jr.; and Standish, M. "Assessing Myocardial Alterations at Autopsy in the Absence of Gross and Microscopic Changes." *Circulation* 37: 218, 1965.

Zugibe, F. T. "Atherosclerosis in the Miniature Pig." In *Comparative Atherosclerosis: the Morphology of Spontaneous and Induced Atherosclerotic Lesions in Animals and its Relation to Human Disease.* Edited by J. C. Roberts and R. Straus. New York: Hoeber Medical Division, Harper and Row, 1965.

Zugibe, F. T.; Conley, T.; Bell, P., Jr.; and Standish, M. "Determination of Myocardial Alterations at Autopsy in the Absence of Gross and Microscopic Changes." *Archives of Pathology* 81: 409, 1966.

Zugibe, F. T. "Relationship Between Chondroitin Sulfate and Collagen." In *Atherosclerosis* in *Le Role De La Paroi Arterielle Dans L'Atherogenese*: Editions du Centre National De La Recherche Scientifique, 15 Qual Anatole-France-Paris Vlle, 1968.

Zugibe, F. T.; Bell, P., Jr.; and Conley, T. "A radiopaque-Plastic Injection Method for Assessing the Coronary Arteries and the Vasculature of Other Organs." *Angiology* 19: 25–35, 1968.

Zugibe, F. T. *Diagnostic Histochemistry.* St. Louis: C. V. Mosby Co., 1970.

Zugibe, F. T.; Conley, T.; Bell, P., Jr.; and Standish, M. "Enzyme Decay Curves in Normal & Infarcted Myocardium." *Archives of Pathology* 93: 308–11, 1972.

Zugibe, F. T. "Detection of Early Myocardial Infarction, A Critique." Proceedings of American Academy of Forensic Sciences, 26th Annual Session, 1974.

Index